GOOD PRACTICES IN PALLIATIVE CARE

Foreword by Dame Cicely Saunders OM, DBE, FRCP
St Christopher's Hospice, London

Good Practices in Palliative Care

A psychosocial perspective

David Oliviere
Middlesex University and Barnet General Hospital

Rosalind Hargreaves
University of Kent at Canterbury

Barbara Monroe
St Christopher's Hospice

ASHGATE

Published by
Ashgate Publishing Limited
Gower House
Croft Road
Aldershot
Hants
GU11 3HR
England

Ashgate Publishing Company
Suite 420
101 Cherry Street
Burlington, VT 05401-4405
USA

Ashgate website: http://www.ashgate.com

British Library Cataloguing in Publication Data
Oliviere, David
    Good practices in palliative care
    1. Social work with the terminally ill 2. Palliative treatment
    I. Title II. Hargreaves, Rosalind. III. Monroe, Barbara
    362.1'75

Library of Congress Cataloging-in-Publication Data
Oliviere, David
    Good practices in palliative care: a psychological perspective
    David Oliviere, Rosaling Hargreaves, Barbara Monroe.
    p. cm.
    Includes bibliographical references and index.
    ISBN 1-85742-396-8 (pbk.)
    1. Pallative treatment – Psychological aspects. 2. Pallative treatment –
    Social aspects. I. Hargreaves. Rosalind. II. Monroe. Barbara. III. Title.
    R726.8.045 1998
    362.1'75--dc21   98-12751

Reprinted 2003

ISBN 1 85742 396 8 (Pbk)

Printed and bound in Great Britain by Biddles Limited, Guildford and King's Lynn.

Contents

Practitioners

Margi Abeles, Family Therapist, London

Mary Baines, formerly Consultant Physician, St Christopher's Hospice, London

Jenny Baulkwill, formerly Principal Social Worker, St Christopher's Hospice, London

Sylvia Bourne, Principal Social Worker, Trinity Hospice

Steve Callus, Bereavement Co-ordinator, Trinity Hospice, London

Catherine Dickens, formerly Head of Cancer Information Service, BACUP, London

Barbara Disney, Assessment and Care Co-ordinator, London Lighthouse

Carol Feldon, Head of Counselling and Social Care, Mildmay Mission Hospital, London

Pam Firth, Senior Social Worker, Macmillan Runcie Day Hospice, St Albans

Janet Foster, Senior Social Worker, St Luke's Hospice, Sheffield

Pat Gardner, Care Manager, Kent Social Services

Stella Hatcliffe, Quality Assurance Advisor, St Christopher's Hospice, London

Frances Kraus, Principal Social Worker, St Christopher's Hospice, London

Wendy Lethem, Home Care Team Leader, St Christopher's Hospice, London

Shirley Lunn, formerly Head of Counselling and Social Care, Mildmay Mission Hospital, London

Joyce Maccabee, Social Worker, Hayward House Macmillan Unit, Nottingham

Pat Mood, Senior Social Worker, Douglas Macmillan Hospice, Stoke-on-Trent

Barbara Monroe, Director of Social Work, St Christopher's Hospice, London

Hardev Notta, Asian Link Officer, Acorns Children's Hospice, Birmingham

Judy Sanderson, Principal Social Worker, St Barnabas' Hospice, Worthing

Jean Simons, Bereavement Services Co-ordinator, Great Ormond Street Hospital for Children NHS Trust, London

Peter Southern, Senior Social Worker, St Bartholomew's Hospital, London

Julie Stokes, Consultant Clinical Psychologist/Programme Director, Winston's Wish, Gloucester

Jane Thomson, Social Work Director, North London Hospice

Joan Towle, formerly Voluntary Services Co-ordinator, Mount Edgcumbe Hospice, St Austell and Vice-chair, Cruse Bereavement Care

Liz Urben, formerly Self-Help and Support Service Manager, Cancerlink, London

Brian Warr, Director of Care Services, Acorns Children's Hospice, Birmingham

Malcolm Williams, Principal Social Worker, St Christopher's Hospice, London

Foreword

Palliative care may begin with symptom control, but in most cases that is only the beginning. Practised as a team, as ideally it should be, palliative care includes every approach that can enable a family to find their own strengths and reach towards the potential for growth that is contained in the situation in which they find themselves. Each person's journey is unique but the expanding practice over the years in addressing psychosocial issues is presented here for both new and experienced workers in this rewarding but challenging field.

The demands of palliative care have been met by developing expanding expertise ever since the original concept of 'Total Pain', with its physical, emotional, social and spiritual components, was presented. The caring concern for dying people, carried out in the few early hospices under a variety of names, has evolved into a network of professional care and expertise, while the workers concerned with the psychosocial and spiritual aspects of management have kept the breadth of need and potential in central focus.

In 1927, Peabody wrote 'What is spoken of as a "clinical picture" is not just a photograph of a man sick in bed; it is an impressionistic painting of the patient surrounded by his home, his work, his relations, his friends, his joys, sorrows, hopes and fears.' This book presents the practice that has led to the development of theory, especially in the thirty years since the opening of the first modern research and teaching hospice. We can hardly better Peabody's description of the people we meet as they face living with a life-threatening illness, whether it be as an isolated individual or as part of a family network. This book will help give confidence in the uncertainty and challenge of each new encounter and also aid in permeating the mainstream from which

Peabody wrote 70 years ago and in which most people will continue to live and die.

Dame Cicely Saunders OM, DBE, FRCP
St Christopher's Hospice, London
October 1997

Acknowledgements

In our professional work there have been many practitioners who have inspired us and they form the background to the experiences recorded in this book. Specific individual practitioners agreed that we might put their work under the microscope and we owe them a huge debt of gratitude.

We would also like to thank our colleagues who made this book possible: in particular Pam Marsh, Joan Roberts and Audrey Shanks for administrative support and Denise Brady, librarian at St Christopher's Hospice, for her patience. Frances Sheldon has been supportive from early planning for this book of practices and Jo Campling's enthusiasm has been sustaining.

We thank our professional colleagues in the Association of Hospice and Specialist Palliative Care Social Workers and the other professional associations who have taught us so much about our own disciplines and how to put multi-professional teamwork to the benefit of those people we are trying to help. We also thank all those from whose openly shared mistakes we have learnt.

Finally we wish to acknowledge both the particular patients, families and carers who talked to us about themselves for this book and the many, many more over the years whose courage in sharing their experiences has been the inspiration for the book and the foundation of our developing practice.

David Oliviere
Rosalind Hargreaves
Barbara Monroe
November 1997

Notes on terminology

The ill person
Patients are referred to as 'the ill person' and in the male gender, unless a specific situation or phrase requires the term 'patient' to be used.

Family
People who are close to the ill person – relatives, partners and friends – or those who have a significant relationship with them.

Carer
People providing informal and unpaid physical and/or emotional care for the ill person whether related by family ties or not.

Professional
The term refers to staff and will sometimes include colleagues working in a voluntary capacity. The professional is referred to in the female gender, unless a specific situation is being described.

Team
Refers both to that group of professionals who are paid and are part of the ill person's helping network, e.g. care staff and care assistants, counsellors, doctors, ministers of religion, nurses, occupational therapists, physiotherapists, psychologists, social workers, and to volunteers.

Introduction

Anything that you have, you can lose,
anything you are attached to, you can be separated from,
anything you love can be taken away from you.
Yet, if you really have nothing to lose, you have nothing.
(Kalish, 1985)

Helping people discover life, while losing it, is the day-to-day stuff of palliative care. This book is about how we can work, intervene and help in situations of loss in the context of practising good palliative care. It focuses on the psychosocial as opposed to the physical aspects of palliative care. It is based on the day-to-day work of experienced colleagues in various palliative care settings.

Whilst the book aims to capture good, sound practices, largely from the mainstream of palliative care, it includes many innovative developments. The book caters for a multi-professional readership of newcomers as well as experienced practitioners in the field who wish to examine actual examples of how others work and to gain new ideas and confirm existing ones.

'The best teachers are patients and families'*

The belief that the ill person and families are the best guides to practice is one commonly held and valued in palliative care. It upholds the palliative care tradition of a person-centred service, of listening well to those with whom we work, and of being led by their needs and at their pace. Even though we might have met several patients before with similar manifestations of symptoms and feelings, practitioners and clinicians in palliative care have always taken care to draw on theory to make sense of the *patient's* experience, rather than just fitting the patient's experience into a theoretical framework. The theory offers an explanation; practice offers the action.

The phrase 'the best teachers are patients and families' may not be literally true but it is a reminder of the interchange and co-operative work that must be undertaken between the ill person and professional staff in order to work

* see Notes on terminology

1

out the way forward in the situation. It moves away from the professional having control, to allowing the patient as much sense of autonomy as is possible. As one experienced hospice doctor put it, 'the patient should preside over his/her own dying' (Lamerton, 1986).

Palliative care has always taught a 'levelling' of patient and professional, based on open verbal and non-verbal communication. Particularly in the area of psychosocial care – as opposed to medical and physical care – the worker does not have a magical set of skills, ready to be used on or for managing needy patients and families. The professional does certainly bring rich knowledge and skills, but essentially she brings experience that will be negotiated with the ill person's wishes, experience and illness. The different elements are blended together to work out the particular consistency of response that is required in any one specific case.

Finally, the phrase 'the best teachers are patients and families' emphasises, not only the uniqueness of the ill person as an individual, but also the uniqueness of the experience – this is a 'once only' for the ill person, family, friends and for the team of professionals and volunteers involved.

What is palliative care?

Hospice and specialist palliative care services aim to promote comprehensive care for those with progressive, advanced disease and a short life expectancy in order to maximise the quality of life remaining, enabling patients to 'live until they die' and includes psycho-social care as well as pain and adequate symptom management. [National Council, 1997a]

An often quoted definition is:

Palliative care is the active total care of patients and their families by a multi-professional team when the patient's disease is no longer responsive to curative treatment. Control of pain, of other symptoms and of psychological, social and spiritual problems is paramount. The goal of palliative care is the achievement of good quality of life for patients and their families. Many aspects of palliative care are also applicable earlier in the course of the illness in conjunction with anti-cancer treatment. Palliative care:

- affirms life and regards dying as normal process;
- neither hastens nor postpones death;
- provides relief from pain and other distressing symptoms;
- integrates the psychological and spiritual sides of patient care;
- offers a support system to help patients live as actively as possible until death;
- offers a support system to help the family cope during the patient's illness and in their own bereavement. [World Health Organization, 1990]

As will be seen from these definitions, the psychosocial aspects of palliative care are totally integrated with all other features of the subject. Every aspect of palliative care contains psychosocial elements:

> The concept of palliative care has broadened over time from 'terminal care' to include the care of those who have a life-threatening disease but are not imminently dying, including people who have recently been diagnosed with advanced cancer and those who have other life-threatening diseases such as multiple sclerosis, motor neurone disease, AIDS, chronic circulatory or respiratory diseases. [Higginson, 1993]

The challenge now for palliative care, more than thirty years since the founding of St Christopher's Hospice, is to redefine its precise role. To what extent have its principles and practices travelled to other specialities and beyond, influencing the physical and psychosocial care of people including the elderly, disabled and bereaved?

Palliative care has opened up discussion and debate on death, dying and bereavement. Should every speciality offer a palliative care element? With the pressures on the public health care sector, is there an ever increasing need for specialist palliative care services? Our view is that specialism is essential to protect and develop core practice standards.

The palliative care approach

The National Council for Hospice and Specialist Palliative Care Services defines the palliative care approach which 'aims to promote both the physical and psychological wellbeing. It is a vital and integral part of *all* clinical practice, whatever the illness or its stage, informed by a knowledge and practice of palliative care principles.' The key principles underpinning palliative care should be practised by all health professionals in primary care, hospital or other settings and comprise:

- Focus on quality of life which includes good symptom control
- Whole-person approach taking into account the person's past life experience and current situation
- Care which encompasses both the dying person and those who matter to that person
- Respect for patient autonomy and choice (e.g. over place of death, treatment options)
- Emphasis on open and sensitive communication, which extends to patients, informal carers and professional colleagues. [National Council, 1995a]

Specialist palliative care services

Services with palliative care as their core speciality are needed by a significant minority of people whose deaths are anticipated, and may be provided directly through the specialist services or indirectly through advice to a patient's present professional advisers/carers (National Council, 1995a).

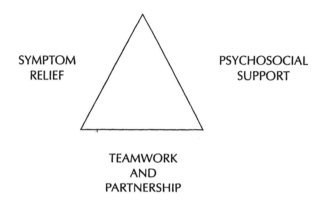

SYMPTOM RELIEF

PSYCHOSOCIAL SUPPORT

TEAMWORK AND PARTNERSHIP

Fig. 1.1   Three essential components of palliative care (Twycross, 1995)

Twycross's triangular diagram highlights the integrated nature of palliative care: any activity in one area has a direct effect on the others. Clearly, uncontrolled pain has implications for teamwork and the ill person's and family's feelings. The areas covered in this book are referred to in the above diagram as 'psychosocial support' and 'teamwork and partnership'.

'Partnership' indicates 'people working co-operatively with a common purpose; it is unlikely to be an equal partnership in the sense that powers, roles and responsibilities are different' (Doel, 1994). Recognition of this element of good care, has been one of the achievements of palliative care.

Practice example

Louis, aged 42, has a brain tumour with extensive secondaries. All the counselling available did not have a positive effect on the pain; alternatively, no amount of morphine or other analgesia blotted out the marital conflict and financial problems he, his wife and two children were experiencing as a result of a failing business and his mood swings. The various aspects of this person's life have to be understood and worked with as a whole.

The nature of psychosocial palliative care

There will be a psychosocial dimension to the work of all disciplines involved in palliative care whether they are: care assistants, counsellors, doctors, home carers, ministers, nurses, psychologists, social workers, therapists or volunteers. The common elements to which we subscribe as professionals in palliative care are:

- total and holistic care
- integrated care
- 'family' as unit of care
- multi-professional teamwork
- best quality of life.

The specific concept of psychosocial palliative care has come to represent an umbrella term covering a number of distinct specialities and areas related to direct work with patients and families, e.g. individual counselling, family work, bereavement care, group work and integrating volunteer roles. It can also involve indirect work, an essential ingredient in helping patient and family, e.g. staff support and multi-professional teamwork:

> Psychosocial care is concerned with the psychological and emotional well-being of the patient and their family/carers, including issues of self-esteem, insight into and adaptation to the illness and its consequences, communication, social functioning and relationships. [National Council, 1997c]

Working in the field of psychosocial palliative care certainly involves a multi-dimensional approach. *Understanding* the phenomena brought by the ill person and his family at different levels – affective (feeling), behavioural (doing) and cognitive (thinking) – and *using* the same dimensions in working with the situation, is essential to good practice. Depending on one's professional training, different models, approaches and therapies are offered.

Key concepts in psychosocial palliative care

Sheldon identifies a number of concepts that have been influential in the development of psychosocial palliative care – attachment, loss, meaning, equity. She asserts that an understanding of them will strengthen the practice of any professional (Sheldon, 1997).

Practising psychosocial palliative care

'To practise' in the field of psychosocial palliative care, as in other special-ties, implies the steady improvement of one's abilities and skills. Professional and volunteer activity involves an amalgamation of values, knowledge and skills. One informs the other. Values form the solid founda-tion upon which knowledge – professional information, theories, models and frameworks – accumulates, which in turn drives the skill at the interface with the ill person and family.

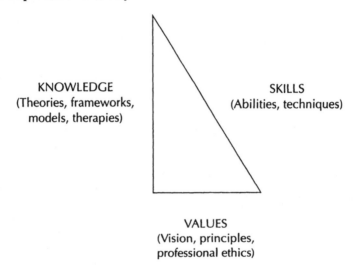

KNOWLEDGE
(Theories, frameworks,
models, therapies)

SKILLS
(Abilities, techniques)

VALUES
(Vision, principles,
professional ethics)

Fig. 1.2   Competence in practice

For example, a secure value base in palliative care of respect for a person's individuality, acceptance and confidentiality will underpin devel-oping knowledge of what terminally ill people experience, the range of psychological states a person lives through and the effects on family dynamics.

Values and knowledge form an essential background to sharpening helping skills in, for example, communicating over sensitive issues or responding to troubled families in order to assist them in pursuing unfin-ished business. At the cutting edge of our work are our practice skills.

Knowledge, skills and values in psychosocial palliative care

These areas of knowledge, skills and values are applicable in other health care specialities and helping activities. They are, however, integral and provide basic means to achieving the aims of palliative care.

- Talking and listening.
- Communicating information.
- Helping people be themselves or to achieve change.
- Assessing the ill person and family.
- Promoting the ill person and carers' rights, strengths and resources.
- Educating the ill person and carer on dimensions of the illness.
- Assisting the ill person and carer to identify issues of concern to them.
- Prioritising and negotiating attainable goals.
- Meeting cultural needs and requirements.
- Helping the ill person and family develop new ways of relating to one another.
- Supporting the ill person, family and carer in their plans.
- Engaging other professionals, agencies and organisations in supporting the ill person and his family.
- Negotiating with the multi-professional team respective roles and responsibilities in partnership with the ill person.
- Helping the ill person and carer adjust to their situation.
- Preparing and supporting families and children over the fluctuating course of illness.
- Intervening in situations of conflict, risk, disadvantage or in specific complex circumstances.
- Assessing and working with bereaved people.
- Working with strong feelings, suffering and intense sadness.
- Sustaining staff and developing one's own practice.
- Facilitating groups.
- Contributing directly to community needs through education.

Day-to-day practice

Day-to-day practice can seem uncertain and testing. However many years we have been practising in our particular role, a new patient and family is a new start and a new challenge. We can mislay that sense of professional competence. This is no bad thing – it ensures a degree of freshness in our approach, openness to what the ill person and family require us to hear, and avoids a total reliance on stereotypical responses and phrases.

In practice, we can easily feel swamped as we experience our professional practice in no way resembling the textbook examples that always seem 'to work'. We do not consciously work just from the secure ground of theory. Much of what we do has been internalised from the theory. Theory and practice can become indistinguishable.

In psychosocial palliative care, the very nature of the work means knowing how to function in shades of grey with uncertainty and ambivalence. Options are frequently less clear-cut than in strictly physical care. The results of interventions are usually less immediate and tangible.

In our own experience, day-to-day work is significantly influenced by how others do the job. Many people's work is directly informed by observing the practices of other, more seasoned practitioners or absorbing the culture of working practices. Some professions have formalised mentoring arrangements in order to maximise observation of practice and modelling of professional skills, behaviour and reflection.

Practice is powerful as a learning tool and we often learn most from our mistakes. Knowing others' working experiences and some of the problems and considerations they have encountered can be supportive. In practice, we do not always 'get it right' and it is important to know of colleagues' struggles to improve their work as well as to acknowledge our own.

Research findings are hugely important by informing theory and practice. However, in reality it takes a considerable amount of time for research findings in health care to affect practice. Research among doctors has shown that 'there is distressing distance between health care knowledge in general and the practices of individual clinicians for validated health care procedures' (Lomas and Haynes, 1987).

'The current emphasis in the United Kingdom on evidence-based health care requires that medical and non-medical professionals ensure that their clinical practice is founded on scientifically derived findings rather than on intuition and ritual' (Hicks and Hennessy, 1997). A number of studies and reports (Hicks and Hennessy, 1997; Royle et al., 1996; Reidenberg, 1996; Higginson, Hearn and Webb, 1996) have indicated that there are big gaps between research and evidence and their integration into clinical practice, for all sorts of reasons. Sometimes practices are even contradictory to the research available (Hicks et al., 1996). Research findings are of little benefit to patients or to society if they do not reach the practitioner or if they are not implemented into practice (Dunn et al., 1994).

Learning from good practices

The practices described in this book have been chosen to cover the range of daily activity in psychosocial palliative care.

In the history of the hospice movement, the development of increasingly sophisticated psychosocial approaches has been secondary to the evolution and research of pain and symptom control techniques. However, colleagues in hospice and palliative care units have been increasingly skilled and inventive in caring for the family, handling difficult emotions, promoting volunteer support, initiating community schemes, assessing bereavement risk and running groups for adults, children and young people.

This book has drawn together in one volume solid, ordinary, professional practices. The collection captures a variety of different settings: in-patient units, day hospices, AIDS facilities, hospital support teams and home care services which provide a good standard of psychosocial palliative care. However, the practices chosen for this book are also being performed in other places and settings by experienced colleagues.

Ill people spend the majority of their illness at home and it is here where much of the psychosocial care takes place, unrecorded and mainly undertaken by relatives, partners, friends and neighbours.

Research on the good practices recorded

The practices described were researched and recorded in a consistent way, obtaining information on:

- What is the context and setting of the practice?
- What is the good practice and why was it necessary?
- What were the key steps in realising the practice?
- What were the obstacles?
- What are the basic principles involved and the resource implications?
- What are the key texts and helpful organisations?

In each chapter, a number of contrasting and complementary practices are described, involving a variety of different settings. A synthesis draws together key points that need considering in the specific area of practice. The format has been modified according to the particular subject of the chapter. There is a degree of inter-connectedness between chapters, for example, there is a clear overlap between 'assessment' and 'working with families'. The research was based on a questionnaire to participants, an in-depth taped interview and written information about the practice.

The practitioners interviewed are among the most experienced in palliative care in the UK and in many cases have been pioneers of their services, combining practice, research and teaching. Presentation of their work reflects the particular style of the practitioner. The more experienced readers will appreciate that as theory and practice become integrated, so does the blend of professional skill and one's personality. This forms part of the richness and diversity of the accounts. The descriptions of practice, therefore, are written in the language of practice. They incorporate, in many cases, several years of building on and testing the theoretical base of the practitioners to a point where strict professionalism and personality become harmoniously integrated in the skills employed.

The research for this book focused on individuals' work, but it is recognised that none of the practices were possible without the active participation of colleagues in the teams in which our participants work. Behind each individual health care professional lies a working group indirectly relating to the ill person and family. As the sister of a patient who died of motor neurone disease put it, referring to the multi-professional team: 'It's like a spider's web ... you take away one of the links and it's gone. For me it was the whole thing knitting together in that cocoon of support.'

We invite you to consider the practices critically and to reflect on questions that need answering should you be wanting to replicate or tailor the practice for your own setting or to develop your own practice.

1 The patient and carer perspective

*'There is only one obvious lesson to learn about other people's grief
– to believe what they say about it'
(Polly Toynbee)*

We begin by considering the issues raised by those receiving palliative care services. These must be the inspiration to which good practice is a response. The patients' comments and ideas were recorded during hospice day-care sessions and from carers whose relative experienced services from primary and secondary health care teams. All were asked to share their experience of both the most and the least helpful aspects of the service they had received from the point at which they realised that a cure for their illness was not possible. The data collected is presented in the form of case studies, recorded in the interviewees' own words, and the practice issues are then discussed in relation to any relevant research findings.

Interview with Helen, a carer

Dad was 84 years old when he was diagnosed as having cancer of the upper stomach. This was in March and he died in the June, three months later. He was having difficulty eating but he had a long history of indigestion and so the family didn't immediately get concerned. Looking back, I think that he might have been undiagnosed for some time. He was constitutionally a strong man who had continued to work as a solicitor into his eighties; he had been treated for glaucoma and in the seventies had had a brain haemorrhage which had been misdiagnosed as a psychological disorder. His period in a psychiatric hospital, being thereafter in his medical records, did I believe, affect the way in which some health professionals responded to him. My mother, also in her eighties, lived with my father in a Welsh rural community. The nearest general hospital was 30 miles away as a result of which there were very highly developed primary health care teams (PHCT)

11

in the area. There were three adult children all with fairly 'high-powered' jobs and none of us living close by. I lived about 250 miles from my parents.

It soon became clear that Dad was seriously ill and he was admitted to the general hospital. The doctor told my mother what the diagnosis was and she telephoned us (the children); we then told my father. We were never really sure if he had ever been told directly. He was given a life expectancy of six months to a year. I was there when a hospital social worker came to see Dad and was distressed to find her very patronising of my mother as the 'primary carer' and also inefficient in following through on what she had agreed to do. I have no reason to suppose that this person was in any way typical of the hospital social work team: I think we were just unlucky in having hit upon an incompetent worker. The experience affected us in that we decided to do everything through my parents' general practitioner (GP).

Our experience of the hospital was pretty negative: no doctors spoke of Dad's condition, only of how soon he could go home. It was clear that, having given one intervention to try to help him eat, they could do nothing further for him and that they needed the bed. No one asked how my mother was going to cope with his care at home. One had a sense that the labels of 'old, cancer and history of psychiatric hospital' were affecting the attitudes of the hospital staff. The GP organised a transfer to the local cottage hospital which was only 10 miles away from home and was less 'high-tec', more 'about basic caring'. The GP visited regularly and was pro-active in contacting the adult children. He had known (and I think, liked) my parents for many years and wanted what was best for them. Whilst we were finding out about our nearest hospice and nursing homes, it was the GP who reminded us: 'That isn't what he wants. He'd be as well staying in the cottage hospital as going to a hospice. He wants to come home.' I realised that the doctor had never discussed alternatives with Dad because he had never wanted anything else except to come home. What we didn't realise at the time was that this particular PHCT was committed to the patient's right to die at home and had policies and services in place to implement domicilliary palliative care; the entire multi-professional team was involved in that commitment, as were any locums appointed.

Dad was now thought to have only a month to live. He wanted to come home and the GP was supporting him in this. He, the doctor, was therefore assessing us, the children, as potential resources to help Dad achieve his wish. Looking back on it, he was very skilled, holding quietly and firmly to his purpose whilst keeping us focused on how we – a partnership between the PHCT and the family – could provide the care Dad would need in order to die at home. I noticed that unlike the hospital, the GP did not identify Mum as the primary carer, though he was careful to include her in all the discussions and planning, checking out what she could and could not do for Dad herself. The problems for us, the adult children, in leaving our own children and work responsibilities to travel to Wales and look after Dad were enormous, but still the GP pushed us to think about how important our decision would be, not just for our parents but for ourselves as we reflected on events later. Eventually we agreed on a plan in which each of the three of us would stay for a week at a time and be the primary carer. I was first on the rota and when my brother brought him home from the cottage hospital, I experienced a sense of panic at the thought of coping with his intimate care needs. The district nurses arrived with him, however, and their 'no-nonsense, down-to-earth' approach, often parodied, was exactly right in helping me overcome this anxiety. Almost before I knew it, I had learned how to empty his urine bag and fit the new one and become proficient at dealing with tubes of one kind or another. Mum had said that she felt perfectly able to care for him for the first couple of days: she, like the rest of us, had had her 'care lessons' and felt confident. As I arrived home the same day, however, the GP telephoned to say that Dad was deteriorating fast and I should return. My two brothers had been contacted and they were also on their way back to our parents' home.

As it turned out, this was the last week of Dad's life and we were all there, one in a nearby B&B, one on the sofa and I slept on the twin bed in Dad's room. I mentioned to the GP that I was afraid that Dad might die whilst I was asleep and he immediately organised for a volunteer sitter to stay in the room so that I could get some sleep. I was amazed that I could actually go to sleep with a complete stranger a few feet away, reading a book, but these volunteers had been so well-prepared for this work: they were unobtrusive, sensitive and tactful and it seemed perfectly natural to have them there. They were only needed for a week but they were prepared to be there indefinitely. We continued to care for Dad during that week, aided 'with a light touch' by the district nurses. We also made sure that Mum got periods of time alone with him so that they could talk. The death when it came was calm and peaceful and all four of us were there. We were all glad that things had been arranged to allow Dad to die at home: it had been profoundly important to him and afterwards, we knew that it had been right for us too.

Interview with Joy, a carer

It was 15 months between the diagnosis of an incurable cancer and Peter's death in hospital. He had been admitted 13 times, five of which were for chemotherapy. It started with very swollen ankles and the GP said at once it could be a symptom of kidney disorder and sent him straight to the hospital out-patients department. He was admitted for tests and at the end of three days, Peter phoned to say that 'the kidney team' had approached him with 'very long faces' and he knew that they 'were going to tell him something awful'. The specialist had explained the problem in 'tremendous technical detail'; the disease was named as 'multiple myeloma' and Peter said that no one used the term cancer, but he was sure that it was. Shortly after I got to the hospital with one of our daughters, a house doctor came over and said 'I've just come to go over it again in case you didn't understand it.' But then, in the next breath, she said to Peter 'You've got an illness called multiple myeloma which is an incurable cancer.' I thought it was good that she recognised that you can't immediately take in news of a serious illness and had come to go through it again, but that stark, single sentence, I don't know, even looking back on it now, if I would say that was the right thing to do. It was a terrible shock. It would have been wrong to keep us in the dark, of course, but I'm still very unsure about what is the 'best' way to break it to the family. When I returned with my other daughter, the haematologist had already spent an hour with Peter, drawing diagrams to answer his questions and grasping his wrist as he said, 'This illness isn't curable, but it's treatable.' That gave us hope that he would at least have some time. It was suggested that because he had kept himself fit and was relatively young, an intensive course of chemotherapy, though it would make him feel very poorly at the time, could give him three or four years of life. Nearly a year later, Peter reflected back on his decision and wondered how he might have fared without the treatment. He hadn't been feeling particularly ill until the treatment started. You wonder about those things and even now, I feel the need to ask the consultant what difference it would have made. The chemotherapy sessions were the worst part of the whole period – for us watching the effect on him and for him, experiencing it. I don't know how much of my negative feelings were coloured by anxiety about his discomfort but we (the family), reacted badly to what we experienced as phoney kindness. The nurse who was fitting the bag of ingredients for his treatment and who was standing some four or five feet away from Peter said 'Was it an awful shock for you? I suppose it must have been.' It was the very first time he had had this treatment and it was traumatic, especially for our daughter. I'm sure the nurse could feel our hostility but we didn't want pseudo-counselling from her: we wanted to feel that she was a competent, accurate nurse who would put the right things in that concoction. There's no reason to suppose that she wasn't, but this style of talking to us really jarred. Then she said to me, 'Do you want to be called Joy? Most of our patients liked to be called by their first name.' I said, 'No thank you.' I was feeling very angry and thinking: why does he have this terrible illness and need to have these horrible things done to him and all these people can do is be artificially charming. We later came to recognise the capability of this nurse but at that time, she got it wrong for us. It all felt insincere and so different from the straightforward kindness of the staff on his original ward.

Over the whole period, Peter was in five different wards and we really felt the difference in the 'culture' between them. One of the 'best' had a very stable, experienced team of nurses and we had confidence that they knew what they were doing and they always took our worries seriously. The ward we felt least confidence in had several nurses who seemed more interested in joking with the less seriously ill male patients than responding quickly to the needs of the very ill. I know that these are impressions based on just a few weeks at a time but they are important to the whole experience of care for the family. Very few of the wards seemed to have enough nurses to cope adequately with helping very weak patients to eat or wash or clean their teeth. I went every day that Peter was in hospital and often did those kinds of things for him. I could accept that a hospital was under-funded and short-staffed and that from time to time, a professional might say something in a clumsy way; we all do that. But I couldn't bear it when they appeared not to care how much someone was suffering, whether it was by laughing and joking when a patient needed something urgently or by saying what they thought were the right words and not having any idea what patients and families were really feeling.

Peter had five sessions of chemotherapy and reacted badly to three of them, with pneumonia twice and shingles after the fifth, so they didn't give him the sixth one. There was a brief period in the early summer when he was at home and spent long periods in the garden; it was idyllic, really. The GP, who had always come immediately we called and often when he was just passing, was always kind and attentive and everyone in that practice was the same. Having people like that in the background, even when Peter was so often in the hospital, gave us confidence. There were only two occasions when I felt at odds with the GP: one was when he tried to talk to me on the way out of the house after a visit and I insisted that we return to Peter's room and discuss it with him. The other was to do with what seemed like his assumption that Peter would go to the local hospice at the end. When he first raised it, I wasn't anywhere near ready to think about that and in any case, I didn't want Peter to go into the hospice; I had visited a friend there and been upset when a nurse had told me that 'they', meaning the staff, thought that it was 'good for patients to see what happens when someone dies', and they appeared not to offer the kind of privacy that I knew I would want for saying good-bye. It was just the one remark but that together with what struck me as choreographed kindness from the moment one entered the foyer, really made me prefer that Peter should die either at home or in the ward where I knew they genuinely cared about him. Looking back, I don't know how I would have coped with him dying at home but in any case it didn't seem to be something which the primary health care team was geared up to. They made sure that we had the district nurses, who were excellent and got us any equipment that would ease Peter's discomfort but everyone seemed to assume that he would die in the hospice. I don't know if Peter refused it because he knew I didn't want it. When I look back on it now, I think that the GP was trying to face me with something I wasn't yet ready to consider. He obviously thought that the end could come sooner rather than later and he saw the hospice as the best place, so he pushed the idea. As time passed, with more hospital admissions, both the consultants were giving us an hour a week to answer questions and explain their thinking about how to keep him going. He was first admitted to a ward where we had never been before but which was very humane and civilised and we had some wonderful quiet moments together, although he was so ill. After a few days however, he was abruptly moved, to my horror, to a ward where I felt that no one had any respect for the patients. Peter was treated very casually as if he were a healthy man in for a minor operation, rather than a very ill man needing a small operation as part of his treatment.

Three things saved my sanity on this ward: the wonderfully warm-hearted 'tea lady', the nice 'newspaper lady' and a visit from the University chaplain who sat with us quietly and then prayed over Peter silently for what seemed like a long time.

To our relief, Peter was then transferred to the [kidney] ward where we knew that they were kind and efficient, and as it turned out, that's where he died. He was in a corner by a window and somehow, we managed to make a private space for ourselves.

On what turned out to be the day he died, I said to a nurse I knew quite well, 'If he's going to die tonight, I will stay.' She comforted me and said, 'Although we know he's very ill, he's not ready to go yet.' I left at 10 p.m. and at 12.15 a.m. was awakened by the phone: it was a senior nurse I knew quite well and she told me that Peter had died. I was alone in the house and started shaking violently. I was very hurt and angry and kept repeating that I'd looked after him for 15 months and had wanted to be with him when he died. She listened patiently, asking who she could get to come and be with me; eventually I was able to respond and our new Rector arrived. I phoned the ward and asked the nurse to make sure that Peter was not moved as we were on our way and wanted to sit with him. The nurse said that the bed was curtained off, there was a soft light on next to the bed and there were enough chairs for us. I was really grateful to know that they had been so thoughtful.

When we went in to see him, he looked absolutely magnificent – like a healthy young man. It reminded me of when I first met him and how he must have looked at Cambridge. He looked triumphant. We sat with him for about two hours. At one point, we went to the nurses' office and drank tea; the nurse told us as much as she could. I said, 'We'll go at ten to four' and we did. We were broken-hearted that he had died and I was bitterly hurt that I hadn't been with him, but when we arrived to see him and to say goodbye, they got everything right and I'll always remember that with gratitude. Something else which was a tremendous help to me was that there was counselling available for patients and relatives and this was of inestimable benefit to me in coping with Peter's illness and his death.

Interview with Elaine

I don't think there can really be a 'good' way to learn that you have an illness from which you may not recover but I do think that there are some ways of breaking bad news which should be avoided. After having had X-rays, the radiologist said, 'Everything's fine but I'd like you to come back for another one, to make sure.' What he could have said quite truthfully was 'There may be something there; the hip looks OK but I'd like to have a look at a different area.' When the urologist saw the subsequent X-rays of the kidneys, he just said, 'That's got to come out.' I was being told that I would have to lose a kidney before I'd been told what was wrong with me. I just glazed over – switched off. The next day I went to see my GP; I told him what had happened at the hospital. He had a sort of smile on his face and said, in what felt like a very patronising way, that everything was going to be all right. He seemed to be puzzled that I should have gone to see him and he was obviously uncomfortable in the situation. I changed my GP immediately and got a woman doctor who somehow found the time for me to talk. It's so important to be listened to, especially at the point where you've just been given that kind of news, even if you keep saying the same thing over and over again. It's necessary, so that you can begin to believe it. If she didn't know the answer to a question, she would say so and her honesty gave me confidence.

I found, though, that even with so much support from my GP, when I came round from the operation, I realised that I hadn't believed it would really happen and I went into shock because I hadn't accepted it. I remember insisting on looking at the X-rays, as if that would mean anything to me or change anything. The nurses were extraordinarily understanding of these bouts of irrationality. I couldn't fault the standard of nursing: it was just very professionally done with genuine kindness.

Three months later, they found more tumours, this time on the second kidney and on the adrenal gland. I had originally found the consultant very abrupt and rather stand-offish but I came to value him for his determination to get the very best treatment possible for me. There were five malignant tumours on the kidney, though I was told that they weren't 'the worst kind'. They were removed at a specialist hospital and then the kidney was monitored. I had heard that the drug Interferon was being used semi-experimentally at that hospital and my local consultant supported my request to try it. A year after the treatment, there was still no sign of any further tumours.

Looking back, the general manner of my consultant did initially increase my anxiety but once I was established as his patient, I felt that he was really committed to my care; he even called at my home one Sunday morning on his way somewhere, just to see how I was doing. What he *did* became much more important than his manner of talking to me.

Probably the greatest difficulty I've had, though, is my family's inability to accept that this illness is as serious as it is and once out of hospital, there was only my GP who could listen to my hopes and fears. It was actually a nurse from the hospital who first told me about the hospice day centre (her husband had cancer and had found it really helpful) and I have found it a tremendous support – being with people who accepted the realities of the situation. In fact, the most invaluable thing about the hospice is that you can say anything and people will know what you mean; you don't have to explain yourself or justify yourself. Another thing is that the staff are there to give you anything they can and nothing is too much trouble. It takes a while to understand and accept that but when life goes on at home as if you weren't ill, it really helps to be indulged in that way. The alternative therapies are part of that: they are things which give your body comfort, important when your body is otherwise not much of a source of pleasure! I've had aromatherapy and reflexology regularly and I have my hair done quite often. There are very few 'minuses' about the hospice day care. I was once patronised by a volunteer who said she enjoyed 'helping poor people' like me and I thought 'It's as if she can't understand that it could happen to her as well.' We have organised entertainment from time to time with local people – concerts and so on; it's not to everyone's taste but it's not compulsory to go, either, so you couldn't really call it a 'minus'. I think that being patronised, whether it's a reassuring 'pat on the head' from a doctor or an insensitive remark from someone visiting, is for me, one of the things I most resent about being this seriously ill. But that's only an occasional experience: hospice day care has made the difference for me between being able to bear things with fortitude and giving up.

Interview with Terry

It took two years from when I first started to feel ill to getting a diagnosis. Finally, I said to my GP 'I still feel as bad as I did when I first came to see you.' He referred me to a neurologist and he had a CAT scan done. They were straight with me from the beginning: all they could do was control the size of the tumour. I've been lucky with my doctors on the whole; I've always been able to get them to have a laugh and a joke with me and I've always managed to get them to be straight with me about how I'm doing and what their ideas are. From a professional point of view, the best doctor was an Asian registrar: he was very clear when he explained things and he had a lovely manner. At the beginning, one or two doctors didn't tell me enough, but I've turned most of them around! I've mainly had chemotherapy; I did try radiotherapy once but it made me feel worse than anything. The tumour goes dormant for a while and then flares up again. It's just got to be kept under control and I think I've done quite well. It's been five years now.

The worst thing about the hospital is the way the consultants do their ward rounds. I really hate it; they come in droves and it feels as if you're some sort of animal – being shown off. You wouldn't mind one or two but sometimes it's nine or ten; I just hate it. You feel so vulnerable when you're lying down and they're standing up. If I can sit up, it's not quite so bad. I don't know why the consultant, at least, can't sit down to talk to the patient. It would make such a difference.

I wasn't surprised when they suggested the hospice. I've just been surprised how long I've been coming here. The hospice home care nurse is very important in my life; she visits regularly and always has time for me to talk – about anything, really. I'm at home on my own for long periods of time; my wife is at work. The district nurse is a lovely woman and she's good at her job but you know she has hundreds of other people to take care of, so I never try to keep her for a chat.

The hospice is where you go to be spoiled rotten! The hospital has done me proud, but it's the hospice that keeps my pain under control and helps me feel that life is still good. I don't lie to them and they don't lie to me, so when I tell them that the pain is too much, I get whatever it takes to keep it down. But it's a place that makes you feel cared about; it also stops me thinking too much about what might happen next. I never ask people what's wrong with them at the day centre. If they want to talk, that's fine but I don't know what's wrong with anyone in here. I don't know if it's an unspoken rule, but that's the way it is. Diversional therapy is important to me; I can make things to sell for fund-raising and I like to do my part. You can choose what you do, thank goodness; I never fancied painting stones, myself! We get some interesting speakers too – on local history, which I never knew anything about.

The main difference you notice between the hospital and the hospice is that they don't have enough staff to care for people the way they should in the NHS. You can see the nurses are worn out, just trying to do the basics; night-staffing is the worst. The patients see what they go through first-hand. It's not right. I think that hospices still have a public image of places you go to die. I know when it was first suggested to me, I was upset because I thought it meant I only had five minutes to go – but it's been five years now and I'm still here! I don't think most people know what goes on in hospices. When our group leaves at half-past three and you're trying to talk to someone, you can't hear them for the laughing. That's what helps me.

The case studies

These accounts are the thoughts and recollections of four people whose experiences of palliative care are either current or recent. As such, they are filtered through strong emotion, both positive and negative: a single remark from a surgeon, nurse or volunteer after a particularly distressing procedure or piece of bad news could become fixed indelibly in the memory as something unforgivable; conversely, a word of kindness in similar circumstances could be received with such gratitude that the person and often, the place, could become forever 'wonderful', brooking no criticism. There is no point or indeed need to look for objective analysis in these accounts: our perceptions of critical life events are bound to contain inconsistencies depending on to whom we relate them and how close in time we are to them. The value of such recollections is that they can sometimes identify the unintended distress caused by professionals when a different phrase or simply sitting instead of standing could have avoided it: they bring home to us in a very personal and poignant way what it felt like to be in that situation as patient or carer and much of what has been recounted resonates with the findings of research and published practice experience.

Breaking bad news

Having the responsibility for giving someone bad news is never easy but in palliative care, where the news is potentially a death sentence, doctors acknowledge it to be one of the most distressing tasks they face, whether it is a hospital consultant, a member of their team or the GP who has to explain the significance of test results. As Elaine commented, perhaps there is no 'good' way of telling someone that they have an illness from which they are unlikely to recover, but there are certainly ways that should be avoided and her experience of hearing the proposed treatment before being given a diagnosis would be one of them. It is a task which 'is often done in an insensitive way, even being delegated sometimes to junior and inexperienced staff' (Doyle, 1996). Not only does the inept breaking of such news cause severe distress and anxiety to the patient, but by undermining trust in the medical team, it can seriously hamper subsequent doctor–patient communication which is a primary source of information essential to effective treatment. As Doyle points out, bad news must not only be broken gently but 'may well have to be repeated several times' to enable the ill person to understand and accept it. Terry had appreciated the way in which the hospital doctors had made the time to break the news with kindness and honesty but even when the news has been communicated as well as it can by hospital doctors, patients will frequently consult their GPs, asking for information which they have already received or hoping for some reassurance that the situation is not quite so bad as has been suggested: this needs to be understood as part of the same, often prolonged and emotionally-charged, process of coming to terms with the implications of what one has been told.

Medical information: carer needs; patient rights

A related issue is that of whose 'property' medical information is. It is now generally accepted that it is the ill person who has a right to the information but it is still not uncommon for doctors to tell a relative even when the patient is perfectly capable of receiving it. The relative may or may not then decide to tell the patient. In the case of Helen's father, the doctor told her mother who told one of the adult children, who then broke the news to him; there was very little delay and no apparent harm to family relationships resulted but it is an issue which requires careful consideration. Family relationships or partnerships can suddenly be threatened by one person having such information about another and any third party would need to have a very intimate understanding of the people involved to be able to make a sound judgement about whether or not it was right to do so. In Joy's case, she made it clear that she wanted nothing discussed except in Peter's presence, firstly because she saw the information as belonging to him and secondly because he would know if she was worried and concealing something. Clearly where the ill person's condition is such that they may be unable to comprehend the information, someone close to them should properly receive it but most people today would regard any information about their health as belonging to them. The patients interviewed for the case studies emphasised their appreciation of doctors who were open in giving information to them as it enabled them to participate in decision making, giving them some control over their lives in a situation where feelings of helplessness tend to dominate. A study by Benson and Britten (1996) following interviews with 30 cancer patients showed that 'most rejected unconditional disclosure of information [to their relatives] without their consent and did not agree that their family should influence what information they [the patient] should be given.' It was very clear that within this small sample, patients valued their autonomy very highly. In an investigation into the quality of care received in the last year of life, Addington-Hall and McCarthy (1995) found that 'relatives bore the brunt of caring for 81 per cent of the sample' (2074) and that 'half the respondents (51 per cent) were unable to get all the information they wanted about the patient's medical condition when they wanted it.' This establishes clearly the experienced need of carers for information about their relative's condition and with some justification, given their responsibilities: it also underlines the tension between the needs of carers and the rights of patients. Citing Randall and

Downie (1996), Sheldon (1997) poses the opposite dilemma for doctors in which the patient makes it clear that they do not want to know any details of their condition, giving *carte blanche* for a relative to be informed about everything: the question then arises, can a seriously ill person have an absolute right to ignorance? Sheldon concludes that unless others are put at risk by it, then the principle of patient autonomy should be paramount.

Emotional aspects of symptom control and carer anxieties

In a recent survey of approaches to palliative care by primary health care teams (Eastaugh, 1996), all participating health professionals thought that the emotional aspect of symptom control was the single most important area of palliative care that needed improving and most acknowledged 'considerable difficulty in dealing with the fear, anxiety and anger experienced by patients in the last phase of their life'. By extension, this would also apply to carers whose levels of distress are often as severe as those expressed by the ill person. As Livesey (1996) comments, 'In the presence of serious illness, however, where there is no respite in the patient's slow, steady decline, it is not unusual for him to ask himself: "Why me? What have I done to deserve this?" ' In considering appropriate responses, Livesey emphasises the value of listening and the dangers of giving advice. In elaborating, he posits two models of interview: the directive and doctor-centred which is closely related to the formal process of history taking and the non-directive and patient-centred which is much less structured, and relies on the patient's initiative. In palliative care, the patient-centred approach, which draws heavily on interviewing skills used in counselling, is generally the more appropriate, particularly when the doctor is faced with powerful emotion.

Places to die and perceptions of hospice

Where one dies often seems to be a matter of chance, depending as much on carer actions toward the end of the ill person's life and the resources available at that point as on anything else. In the review of the Registrar General on Death in England and Wales 1992, cited in Field, Hockey and Small (1997), the mortality statistics (general) showed that out of 558,313 deaths 54.5 per cent died in an NHS hospital, 18.5 per cent in communal establishments (which included hospice deaths), 22 per cent in their own home and four per cent in other circumstances. In the first study undertaken in the United Kingdom reporting patient preferences about places of terminal care (Townsend et al., 1990), 84 patients agreed to be interviewed and 59 stated a preferred place of final care: of these 34 expressed a wish to die at home given existing circumstances, twelve to die in hospital, twelve in a hospice and one elsewhere. After their death, it was found that of the 34 people who wished to die at home, 17 actually did so, whereas of the 32 patients who died in hospital, 22 had said they would prefer to die elsewhere. It was also found that had circumstances been more favourable many more patients would have preferred to die at home. Townsend concluded that 'with a limited increase in community care 50 per cent more patients with cancer could be supported to die at home, as they and their carers would prefer.' Hinton's 1994 study cited in Sheldon (1997), however, does suggest that both patient and carer preferences may shift toward in-patient care as death becomes imminent.

Place of death was an issue for both Helen and Joy though their situations were very different. Helen's father had expressed to his GP a strong prefer-ence to die at home. The adult children's first response, however, had been to seek information about the nearest hospice and nursing homes but were reminded by the GP that this was not what their father wanted. It was in fact the GP's very positive attitude towards deaths at home and a commitment to meeting his patient's wishes, which ensured in this case that no alterna-tive was seriously considered. In contrast, Joy's impression was that, although she had been well supported by Peter's GP and the primary health care team during his periods at home, there was an underlying assumption that Peter would eventually go to the local hospice. In the event, kidney failure precipitated a final admission to hospital and Peter was still seeking medical interventions which might give him a little longer. At this point, Joy and Peter's preference was that he should be on one of the wards in which they had previously experienced much genuine kindness from the nursing and medical staff. Joy felt afterwards that it had been a matter of luck related to the availability of beds which had enabled this to happen.

The two patients who were attending their nearest hospice day care at the time of the interviews were not asked directly if they expected to die in the hospice but it was clear from their positive attitudes to the staff that they would, at that point, wish this to be the case. They had however both under-gone a change of attitude toward hospice care since it had first been suggested. Terry appears to have accepted a hospice referral without reser-vation, probably because he didn't expect to live very long and he did not have any great expectations of it. Elaine had accepted hospice day care as a source of emotional support at a time when her family was in total denial of the seriousness of her condition and she received the support in full measure. The day-care facilities, apart from offering pain and symptom control, provided two positive experiences which were frequently referred to by the patients: the first was a range of therapeutic activities, varying from place to place, but including aromatherapy, reflexology, massage, a variety of diversional therapies, jacuzzi and hairdressing; their value was expressed as giving comfort to bodies which were 'giving out' and the pleasure of being 'spoiled' or indulged. The second experience often mentioned was the opportunity for a laugh. This was explained as either simply making one 'feel better' and by another person as recognition that one does not suddenly lose one's sense of humour because one has not got long to live. Someone else said his friends and family seemed to think that it wasn't right to make a joke in his presence and that his day centre was the only place he felt he could enjoy a laugh. Dean (1997) reviewed the place of humour and laughter in palliative care and found that there were well-established benefits for both patients and staff, not least for the former in terms of pain reduction in response to endorphin release. 'Joking in the face of death', Dean concluded, 'can serve as a protective armour against personal vulnerability.' Both patients interviewed for the case studies provided glimpses of this, even if the humour was wry and retrospective: Elaine recalled that on being informed in very serious tones by a consultant that he could provide her with treatment which would 'prolong her active life,' all she could think of for a few moments was that he intended to offer her a diet of dog food, the slogan for which he had unconsiously used. Despite the demonstrated benefits of humour and laughter in palliative care, the dangers are obvious: one person's idea of what is funny may be wholly unamusing to another; relatives of a person in severe pain or in their very last hours may feel affronted by laughter nearby. Thus great sensitivity and discretion should be used by staff in evaluating advantages for some against potential distress for others.

The issues discussed here briefly are by no means exhaustive but their importance to the patients and to carers emerged clearly from the interviews. A commonly accepted belief is that palliative care patients are probably too ill to wish to take part in research studies and this may be true for some. The Townsend study referred to earlier, however, in which 86 per cent of those approached agreed to take part and of whom 83 per cent died during the study, would seem to contradict the accuracy of that general assumption. Not to *offer the opportunity* is perhaps the ultimate in a patronising attitude.

2 Assessment

'Assessment should never be done to someone but with someone.'
(Oppenheim, 1998)

Assessment begins with a psychosocial study about the ill person and his circumstances with the purpose of securing as much information as is relevant to understanding the situation. Assessment gives an informed position from which to work. It helps form an opinion and it never ends – assessment is ongoing.

The main focus of work early on in our contact with the ill person and family, is assessment, that is, obtaining a picture of their situation. However, it must never remain a 'snapshot' when what is needed is the video. Assessment must always be a regular component in our work (Lukas, 1993).

In specialist palliative care, as the National Council for Hospice and Specialist Palliative Care warns: 'The anxiety and existential doubt of the dying patient and the grief of those close to them are normal and should not be necessarily pathologised, nor should it be assumed that professional intervention is always appropriate' (National Council, 1997c).

'Assessment' has become a popular term and a key to accessing services. With the implementation of the National Health Service and Community Care Act 1990, there has been much emphasis on general assessment of need within communities and specific assessments of whether newly referred patients are eligible for particular services.

Taking time to assess is imperative if one is not going to be drawn into the strong emotion surrounding the ill person and propelled into inappropriate 'doing'. One needs to take time to listen and agree with the ill person and family the work to be achieved. Assessment provides an opportunity to discuss some areas on which to concentrate and to aim, so that the intervention can be *purposeful*: 'It is important for the psychological and emotional state of both patient and carers to be assessed at an early opportunity so that appropriate levels of support, and treatment when necessary, can be offered' (National Council, 1997c).

Assessment entails developing an understanding of the ill person and their needs, wishes and views and linking these with what can be offered

25

and skills available. It is through the process of thorough assessment that one builds up a working relationship with the ill person and family, locating areas of concern and identifying areas for change.

Assessment challenges all our knowledge, values and skills in working in an integrated way. Assessment and intervention are closely intertwined. Whilst carrying out the process of assessment, as professionals, we are simultaneously intervening in the person's life, for example, building up a therapeutic relationship with the ill person and family, engaging them in a helping process, allowing them to feel safe and comfortable, communicating interest and respect, carving out time to allow their anxieties to surface. Thus, there is a catalytic effect of assessment. Much of palliative care is very short term and we frequently assess and intervene within one or two sessions.

This demands analysis and clear thinking on the issues presented whilst remaining spontaneous and empathetic. The key element is working out with the ill person and carer what is uppermost in their concerns. This is a complex process frequently involving conflicts of interest and priorities between those involved, e.g. parent and adult son or daughter, at a time when usual coping mechanisms and emotions are frequently distorted and when so many taboos result in a family requiring considerable initial help in naming the issues at stake before being able to identify needs.

This chapter will introduce the process of assessment and examine the elements that comprise good assessment by considering the work of practitioners, giving three different accounts of assessment: in a hospital palliative care team, a hospice and a specialist hospice for people with AIDS. This will clarify the content and process of assessment in contrasting settings. It will conclude with a framework for psychosocial, holistic assessment.

Assessment is part of a process:

- gathering information
- making an informed assessment
- agreeing goals/priorities with ill person/carer
- planning
- intervention
- review and evaluation.

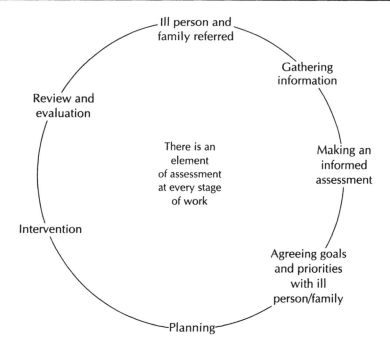

Fig. 2.1   The cycle of assessment

Psychosocial assessments in palliative care

In assessing the individual we need to establish what changes the illness has wrought as well as who they are. We need to know how their life has changed since the illness and who or what currently supports them. We need to understand their reaction to the illness and its implications for them. We need to identify any practical or emotional unfinished business they may have. Assessing practical issues will lead us on to values and beliefs. Does the individual see their illness as a punishment? How have they dealt with crises in the past? [Monroe, 1993b]

Family assessment in palliative care is also seen as important:

In order to assess the strengths and difficulties of a family and its members, we need to understand how it works. We must discover the normal patterns of communication, support, and conflict in the family, and the extent to which they have been disrupted by illness ... The history of the current family and their individual experiences within their previous families will be significant factors in their ability to cope with the present crisis. [Monroe, 1993b]

Monroe asserts that an assessment requires four perspectives: the individual, the family, physical resources and social resources.

Randall and Downie raise the moral and ethical issues evident in having to question individuals and families about personal and sensitive information. This is intensified by the difficulty in justifying the benefit of these psychosocial practices which are difficult to evaluate by research (Randall and Downie, 1996).

Whilst carrying out assessments, therefore, one has to be mindful of the reasons for requiring substantial amounts of information and the impact this may have on those subject to assessment. In good practice, we have to be careful to agree with the ill person and family, the reason for our enquiries, to know that they consent and to check with them their reactions as the assessment progresses. This also involves explaining the nature of grief and giving clear permission for individuals and families not to have to talk about areas they prefer to keep private.

Assessment in a hospital, multi-professional palliative care team (support team)

Peter Southern, Senior Social Worker, Palliative Care Team, St Bartholomew's Hospital, London

The setting is a multi-professional team in a long-established teaching hospital in the city of London. The team comprises a part-time consultant, senior registrar, senior nurse specialist (team leader), nurse specialist, administrator/secretary and senior social worker. The team has no in-patient beds of their own but referrals must come from medical teams. The area covered consists of a number of London boroughs where there exists a high incidence of poverty, unemployment and poor housing, within ethnically very diverse communities. The team is working within a hospital culture where distress is sometimes seen as negative and a not uncommon view is that 'crying and angry people have to be stopped'!

The good practice

Psychosocial assessment takes place within a hospital support team setting: family assessment with particular emphasis on the ill person as part of a network, with a recognition of the needs of children. Good assessment begins long before face-to-face contact with the ill person and family and involves time spent assessing the referral. The team adopts the following process.

The team discussion

The team discusses the referral and makes an initial assessment of who needs to be involved. The nurse or doctor would usually undertake the first part of the assessment process unless it was clearly evident that there were social problems.

Liaising with colleagues

As much information as possible is obtained from the medical and nursing staff of the referring teams, listening to colleagues' concerns and where they consider the palliative care team can be most effectively involved. A history is taken from the medical notes.

Reflecting before reacting

Time is spent considering if it is appropriate for the palliative care team to become directly involved with the ill person/family or whether the team can work indirectly by helping the staff to do the work. This is particularly relevant when teams are working in a consultative capacity and also performs an educative and confidence-boosting function.

The team considers the appropriateness of a local hospice or palliative care team being introduced near the home of the ill person. Working collaboratively and deciding respective roles are important tasks to achieve.

Practice example

Mr M., an elderly Bengali man, was referred to the palliative care team with terminal cancer. The message on referral was that the family were uncooperative, rude, aggressive and difficult. Staff were distressed and concerned for the patient. The family was not communicating with staff.

Once the team met the patient, it was clear that he spoke little English but was giving instructions to his sons to discharge him. The son was very anxious to please his father and to respect his final request and this was of prime importance to the family.

The ward had overlooked the importance of addressing basic communication with a person whose first language is not English. With an interpreter involved, it was possible to appreciate the patient's fears and anxieties, give expression to them and for the ward staff to assist the family in helping their father. The palliative care team's role was primarily in establishing communication.

Team members' own responses to referrals

How patients make *us* feel needs to be borne in mind in forming opinions and in carrying out assessments. Are we making judgements based on whether the ill person makes us feel angry, protective or frustrated? We need to be aware of the influence of our developing relationship with the ill person/family and how this impacts – positively or negatively – on the outcome of our assessment, e.g. do we like them? How do we react if we do not share their values and attitudes towards, e.g. honesty, the role of women, the health service? Do we feel that what has happened to them is particularly 'unfair'?

Use of genograms/family trees

Genograms or family trees are used regularly in complex situations. This encourages people to open up areas of concern and helps professionals see patterns and perceive family conflicts.

The genogram is a useful tool for providing information and further information flows from the discussion of people and relationships identified. It is an assessment and a therapeutic tool and puts a safe framework around helping people talk about their emotions.

The use of the genogram is a good example of where the process of assessment and intervention can be closely interconnected, particularly where one has one or two sessions with a patient/family. (See below for description of genograms/family trees.)

Entry in notes

Communication among the professionals involved is an essential element in assessment when much information is being gathered, plans are being formulated and roles being identified. One needs to communicate succinctly the assessment plan and engage colleagues as part of it.

The process of writing down one's observations firms up one's thinking around assessment.

Questions in formulating assessment

In the process of making an assessment the following questions should be asked:

1.   What has prompted the referral? Why now? What for? What is the person making the referral expecting from the team? Are we seeing the person/family through someone's else's eyes?

2. What is the ill person/family's understanding of my role? What have they been told about the team? e.g. do they have written material, are they specifically expecting pain control only?
3. Where is the patient in treatment? How are they today?
4. Have I made it clear why I've come and what the referral was about? How much time have I got?
5. Have I listened to the *patient's* assessment of what his needs are, whilst keeping my own checklist of what I think the difficulties and issues might be?
6. Have I been sensitive to the non-verbal exchange as well as to the verbal communication from the ill person/family, e.g were they *saying* one thing and was I left *feeling* another? Analysing one's own emotional responses and taking the temperature gauge of one's own feelings provides useful assessment information.
7. Have I explored the issues important to the ill person/family?

Content of psychosocial assessment

The following factors are considered during assessment:

- Illness   The history of illness and the understanding the ill person possesses of what is happening, as well as their emotional and psychological response. How the illness is affecting the ill person physically and his ability to carry out his role, viz. parent, mother, lover, etc.
- Family   Family history; who is around; where; how important are they; how supportive are they?
- Life stresses   What is happening regarding money, jobs, housing, children, sources of support (schools, churches, friends, clubs)?
- Hopes and fears   What is the worst thing that can happen? Plans? Disappointment? Unfinished business? What does the ill person still wish to accomplish?

The value base underpinning assessment

Peter Southern emphasised that a sound value base is seen as essential in guiding the work of assessment:

- Valuing and respecting the person and their uniqueness and diversity
- Non-judgemental attitudes from the professionals
- Confidentiality
- Reliability
- People have their own resources and these should be maximised
- Therapeutic value of listening empathetically to someone's 'story'.

Practice example

Mrs A., 30-year-old white woman with cervical cancer originally diagnosed in 1995. Received treatment with chemotherapy and radiotherapy.

Mr A., 32-year old builder of Asian origin (parents from India); his family
live nearby. Children:

- Girl, 13 – daughter of Mrs A., from a previous relationship; little
  contact with her father
- Girl, 11 – just started senior school
- Boy, 8
- Girl, 5 – just started primary school.

Mrs A.'s parents live round the corner. Father works full-time; mother has
been helping her daughter with child care since the diagnosis. Mrs A. has
a younger brother who is married.

Difficulties in assessment

The following illustrates the difficulties encountered in assessment.

Mrs A. lives some distance away, i.e. 30 miles, from the hospital where the
assessment is being undertaken. Relatives and friends visit only occasionally. Assessment based on contact with patient only.

Initially Mrs A. was in hospital for very short periods of two days for
chemotherapy. She had numerous out-patient appointments and received
radiotherapy as a day patient. Treatment at this point was curative, although
with the likely outcome of recurrence within the next 1–2 years.

As a result of being on different wards and clinics, and seen by different
nursing and medical staff, the building of relationships with hospital staff
was problematic.

In addition, Mrs A. was suspicious and understandably 'ignorant' of the
social work role. She developed more understanding and a better relationship with social workers following the provision of practical help, i.e. information about local social services in relation to possible childminding as
well as a grant to cover travel costs.

Regarding her personality and coping style, she appeared isolated and
frightened when in hospital. This led to withdrawal 'on a surface level'. The
patient did not want to 'talk'. It was important to respect her coping style
even if it made it difficult to build up a clear picture for assessment
purposes.

Outcome

Mrs A. was re-admitted to hospital 18 months after treatment with recurrence plus secondaries and received palliative care only. She experienced major relationship difficulties with her husband. Mrs A. died three months after this admission after a difficult terminal phase: the marital relationship had become increasingly conflictual, the children had little chance to communicate with their mother and many were concerned about their needs.

Mrs A.'s family of origin was in turmoil. A previous death of a child (the patient's brother) magnified the emotional pain these parents were experiencing and the distress in the situation.

Clearly the practice limitations and dilemmas are evident in carrying out a psychosocial assessment in this situation and sometimes professionals only have permission to undertake partial assessments.

A family-based approach to assessment

Judy Sanderson, Principal Social Worker, St Barnabas' Hospice, Worthing, West Sussex

The setting

Judy Sanderson undertakes psychosocial assessment with whole families as part of a multi-professional team in an established hospice for adults. The hospice provides 25 beds, day and home care in an area with a high proportion of the population over retirement age. Few ethnic minority groups exist within the local population. People are generally referred to the hospice further down the treatment line when other colleagues may have already offered them psychosocial help.

The good practice

A flexible approach to needs assessment with the ill person and family, which is patient-led and professional-guided, is adopted. It is an approach that acknowledges age, culture, gender, sexual orientation, family dynamics, individual choice and the different systems which interact in the patient's life.

In this approach to assessment, Judy Sanderson emphasises its holistic nature, i.e. not just focusing on one aspect of a patient and family's need. The basic approach requires standing back and looking at the family from various viewpoints, internally as well as externally, and to consider the impact for the local community in which the ill person lives.

Assessments do not have tidy beginnings. Psychosocially, one can become involved at any stage during the illness. Quite often, by the time the ill person is referred to the hospice, there will have been considerable involvement and information. Nurses and doctors in palliative care are generally quite skilled at identifying areas of need and involving colleague psychologists, counsellors and social workers for more specific assessment and intervention.

Practice example

Mr D., husband of a patient, aged 60 years, had sent a letter to a home care sister indicating what sounded like a 'suicide pact' with his wife. The social worker was immediately involved and, using her previous experience in the mental health field, she made an assessment, liaising closely with the home care sister and joint working with the general practitioner.

What emerged was the extent of this man's own need and a previously unknown history of severe depression (he had a different GP from his wife). In addition to appropriate medication, brief intensive support was offered him which enabled him to cope in the short term, whilst longer-term support networks could be put in place.

Identifying the need for psychosocial assessment

It is important to recognise the situations that call for psychosocial assessment:

- Physical symptoms are causing psychosocial distress
- Vulnerable family members are involved, e.g. children, grandchildren, those with learning disabilities or psychiatric illness or with a severe mental health history
- Where the family has experienced other recent losses or has multiple problems, such as poverty, isolation and are likely to require additional support after the death
- Where a more specialist input is required from a suitably experienced colleague.

Process of assessing

Be aware of the family's frustration at having to repeat background information they may have given to several professionals at earlier stages. In making an assessment and becoming involved in observing and gathering information, one must be clear about the *purpose* of the assessment and of what one is being asked to do in making the assessment, e.g. relieve the depression, reduce the denial, make arrangements for a nursing home.

Invest time in sharing ideas and mingling perspectives as a team

Speak to as many team members as possible, collate information and consider aspects which 'jump out at you'. Different facets strike different professionals and that is the richness of a multi-professional look at referrals.

This process generates hypotheses about what may be happening in the family. Explore these hypotheses with colleagues.

Practice example

M. family: The nursing staff were very concerned as an 11-year-old daughter of a male patient and ill wife, was said to be increasingly delinquent. All her behaviour was assessed in terms of delinquent behaviour. The social worker hypothesised that, with two sick parents, this behaviour was a means of showing her reaction to her parents' illnesses. She had been found trying to drive the family car! An exploration with the girl revealed that she was worried about her Dad not eating anymore and she wanted to find 'a really nice restaurant' which she thought was at some distance, in order to tempt him.

As the ongoing assessment continued, it became apparent that there were many longstanding difficulties within the family and that these needed to be addressed within the context of the parents' illness. Liaison with social services, GP, schools and a psychiatrist was important in recognising the extent and complexity of the problems whilst continuing to acknowledge the pain and grief that this girl was demonstrating.

On first interview listen carefully and record

Note points that puzzle you and aspects which can be explored later. Many aspects in an early interview 'don't add up' and need thinking over. Assessment is not an activity you do just once – it is ongoing – so you do not have to tackle all the issues within one interview.

Use of self-knowledge

Understanding of one's own reactions, of one's effect and impact on others is essential in understanding the needs of others. We need to look at our own

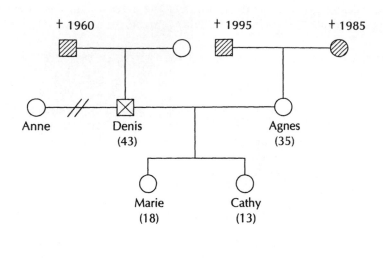

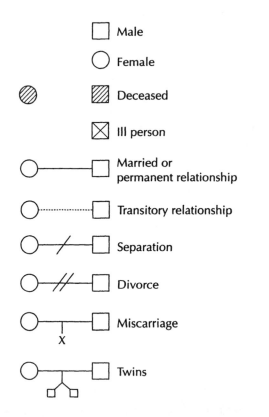

Fig. 2.2   Family trees – an assessment and a therapeutic tool

'cupboards', our own inner world, as this will inform our practice. For example, if I am in great denial over professional staff never acting inappropriately, then it is easy to make assumptions and this will affect my perceptions and the assessment. If I am overcritical of 'men', 'women', of gay or lesbian people, then my attitude will influence the outcome of assessment.

We, our work and our attitude and that of our colleagues, affect the dynamics of a situation. We need to develop our insight. A colleague intervening or discharging a patient may also have an effect on us and our attitude.

Family trees and ecomaps

A family tree helps us gather information as well as discuss significant people and happenings in the family. Family trees illuminate the past living in the present. A family tree clarifies intergenerational relationships among family members, i.e. the influence of the way the family has experienced death or the influence of previous relationships on current family functioning.

An ecomap shows the relationship of the ill person/family to their environment, a map of their territory. The use of lines connecting different parts of the map can clarify interrelationships, isolated people, 'unfinished business' in terms of the ill person's relationships. As with family trees, the person's history emerges in a more concrete way when viewed on an ecomap, and the family remains in control of the material they disclose.

Using an ecomap with a family is a means of empowering a person or family member, for example, a child, to tell you about the people they are close to, where they receive their support and the relationships with the various health and social service agencies who are involved with them.

Use of materials and activities in assessments with families

A range of materials and activities are regularly employed as exploratory techniques (Congress, 1994) in order to engage patients and families in conversation about how they view their situation, their needs and their feelings. Stories, art work, outings, family trees and ecomaps are all ways of recording information, identifying issues, deciding priorities and finding the right medium for work with the individual and family. The activity must be *purposeful* and *understood* by the family. The aim of your intervention always needs to be made clear.

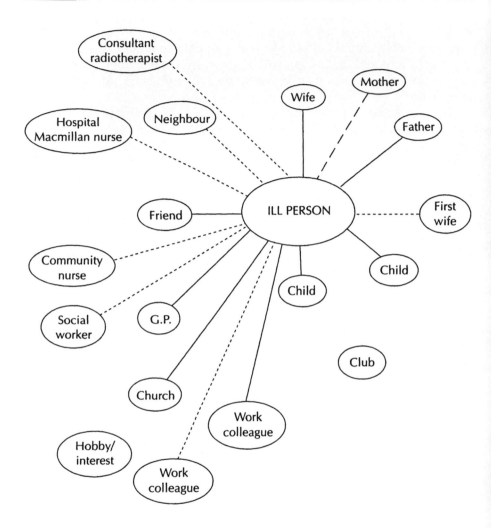

Place ill person or family towards centre of ecomap
• Locate important people or organisation
• Draw lines between circles according to type of
  connections that exist

——————— Strong connection

········· Weak connection

— — — - Stressful connection

Fig. 2.3   Ecomaps – identifying networks

Practice example

A woman of 50 with a short prognosis was very distressed as her family continually maintained an unnatural cheerfulness. The social worker suggested a family meeting and her husband, as well as two adult children, met together with the social worker. It was vital to clarify the purpose of the meeting and to reassure the family that they were meeting to see how they saw the present situation. They had 'to be given permission' to be themselves. Each family member was able to explore the reasons for their behaviour together; for the first time changes became possible. Each contributed openly and significantly to the issues under discussion and agreed that they had felt safe enough to cry, shout and behave as they felt. Tension was reduced and the patient was able to relax, reducing her need for pain control. She said she felt more at peace.

Involvement of other carers

Sometimes other carers, e.g. home carers, escorts (hospital or day centre transport), with the ill person's permission, have much information and helpful observations to contribute to giving a fuller picture of the situation. Make maximum use of the available information, bearing in mind that it has been filtered through others' perceptions.

Summarising diagrammatically

Patients and professionals have very limited time and the use of family trees (Fig. 2.2) and ecomaps (Fig. 2.3) can provide a fast, efficient, focus for work. These methods can help anchor the realities for the ill person and family at a time when life can seem out of control. There are variations in compiling ecomaps and family trees; the style is determined by the family involved. By empowering the ill person or family to tell us about the people they are close to, where they receive their support and the relationships with the various agencies involved with them, ecomaps and family trees enable the family story to emerge in a more concrete way and the family remains more in control of the material they disclose.

Ecomaps and family trees tell us much about family dynamics. Who is not prominent on the drawing or people who are deceased, all add to the understanding of the family and the ill person's place within it. If it is appropriate to invite different members to complete their own ecomaps, the variety of support systems and relationships become visible.

Dialogue with family

Assessment is not a singular act: all work has an assessment component. Part of the process of assessment is clarifying with the ill person and family, 'today, what is most important to you?' This gives control to the ill person and family to include on the agenda for discussion what is important to *them*. It ensures a family-led approach to assessment and communicates to the family that we see them as partners. It is essential to convey that 'your perception and our perception of your needs may change; we can work together.'

Assessments are therapeutic: by undertaking an assessment, the professional is already engaging the family at a deeper level. Explore what is acceptable – culturally, spiritually, intellectually and socially – for the family. Find out what is 'normal' for this particular family as this could put communication patterns, and previous and current relationships into quite a different context. One must cover any practical areas of concern: employment, housing, money, child care, fears after death. Identify any links and relationships in the community that are significant, e.g. schools, churches, clubs.

Dialogue with the multi-professional team

Report your observations and assessment to whoever in the multi-professional team asked for your involvement and with those working in a key relationship with patient and family. Be sensitive and non-threatening to colleagues about your work. You are only *part* of a team and it is essential you work collaboratively, not in competition for disclosures or importance.

Discussion with colleagues over the assessment process opens opportunities for co-working, however short-term, over specific issues. Multi-professional team meetings are about picking up information, signs, asking questions and making suggestions, even when one does not have direct contact with the patient and family.

A patient-focused approach to assessment

Shirley Lunn and Carol Feldon, Head and Deputy Head of Counselling and Social Care, Mildmay Mission Hospital, London.

The Mildmay Mission Hospital is a 42-bed palliative care unit in east London for people with AIDS. It offers rehabilitation and respite care, long-term and terminal care, London-wide. Thirty beds are in the main residential unit, whilst a twelve-bed family unit can house whole families. Several family rooms are available. The counselling and social care department comprises five counsellors and social workers plus one art therapist. Part of the complex is a day centre for adults and a nursery for children with HIV/AIDS. Staff have worked with over two thousand patients since opening and have had extensive experience of assessment within this more specialist setting.

Common features of the care of these patients are: shared care with acute centres; patients whose conditions fluctuate, and where a terminal phase is less clearly definable. Active treatment is frequently continuing alongside palliative care, with the ill person moving between hospice and an acute centre.

Patient-focused care

The unit offers not so much patient-directed care but a patient-focused approach to care. Although one cannot generalise about people referred, in the late 1980s those referred were frequently gay men very much more in control of their lives, often able to articulate their needs and knowledgeable about their rights to services. They clearly wanted to be involved in their care.

The patient population has now shifted with many more drug users, people from the African continent or people with very chaotic lifestyles. Many patients with challenging behaviour have needed more structure. Many of those from the African continent culturally find 'patient-directed care' in the doctor–patient relationship, anathema and sometimes burdensome.

When the ill person is admitted he is told about the various parts of the service and given a set of leaflets describing them. Admitting doctors are trained to offer the new patient the menu of what is available: chaplaincy support, counselling, day care, dietary care, medical care, nursing care and so on. Value is placed on the initial 'assessment', therefore, being carried out by the ill person. A screening or 'prioritisation' process is undertaken by the ill person himself. An interview with the doctor or nurse helps the person decide which parts of the 'menu of care' they wish to receive. This approach clearly gives as much decision making as possible to the patient in controlling which professionals should interact with him. It works on the basis that the ill person's motivation to make good use of the particular service is maximised if he has decided to access the service.

The multi-professional team meets four mornings per week and the doctor presents the patient's preferences for involving the various parts of the service. If the main reason for admission is psychological, for example, a mother with two children admitted and there is concern about the children's welfare, or admission has immediately followed diagnosis, or in situations of psychological distress, then the counselling department becomes the key department and ensures people are seen within three days at a maximum.

Preparation for assessment

Preparation for assessment is as important as actually doing the assessment. In preparing to assess, counsellors read all the patient's notes, recognising that they are making some assumptions. They make a paper assessment of the person and their circumstances.

The counsellor initiates a discussion with ward staff and particularly the patient's named nurse in order to hear how they see the ill person and his needs. This initial discussion allows the counsellor to establish, 'what is a good time of day' to see the ill person. Many young patients, for example, prefer to sleep until late in the day.

Information

In assessing and gathering information, particular care is taken to preserve confidentiality, meticulously checking with the ill person what information can be shared with the team. The practitioners interviewed expressed the view that in the field of palliative care generally, too much is often passed on and that it was important to allow the ill person some control over information about themselves. Sometimes just the area of work is communicated to the team, e.g. 'coping with a violent relationship' without describing the content and details.

Trust

Forming a good relationship of trust, although basic, is essential. Of course, different professionals will use different techniques to help the ill person and family to feel 'safe and comfortable'.

It would seem that this approach to assessment particularly allows the ill person to bring issues to the agenda for discussion. Counsellors engage the person in defining how they are coping emotionally and in considering the illness and its consequences realistically. Concerns regarding family and friends are clarified and specific assessment (e.g. for home support) is made as necessary by the appropriate professional.

A planned assessment format enquiry into key areas of a person's life is not adopted but instead a strong belief in 'starting where the person is'. This particular form of assessment asks the question 'what about the areas that the person has not thought to raise or see as relevant but which could be emotionally charged or problematical?' However patient-focused, the professional has a role in knowing that there could be other areas of concern and for 'listening behind the words'. It also overcomes the problem of people being labelled and defined by the previous stories which accompany them, e.g. 'difficult', 'erratic', 'dependent' – rather than allowing them to be different at different stages of the illness.

Part of the aim of the assessment period is creating a relationship of trust where the ill person and family can return for further discussion.

Practice example

Ross, a 28-year-old man, had been denying he had AIDS and the nursing staff became extremely concerned as he was talking of an arranged marriage. They felt strongly that his wife-to-be would be put at risk.

The counsellor met him and needed to build a relationship and listen to his history of being subjected to torture before further assessment work could be done. She discovered that a marriage had not in fact been arranged but that Ross had talked of wanting a relationship as there were expectations placed on him by his family to have an arranged marriage.

Tension arose between the counsellor and other members of the multi-professional team. The dilemma faced by the counsellor was that other members of the team felt very strongly that in view of Ross's 'denial', the issue should be forced in terms of information about his diagnosis. However, Ross was very wary of professionals as he had been a political prisoner in his country of origin and needed time to build up a relationship of trust with staff before he could begin to acknowledge and accept his diagnosis.

Care plan

By day four of a new patient's admission, a care plan is made by the multi-professional team. These are reviewed and redrawn during the period of admission, hence involving reassessment. Following discharge, a patient is reviewed within three days in order to consider any necessary changes for the next admission.

Overview of assessment

Making an assessment is about creating a safe relationship, respecting the patient and family and structuring a comfortable experience to allow material to emerge. 'Everybody is in the frame', Shirley Lunn insists, 'although one is interviewing the ill person, one is aware of the needs of parents, partners, work issues, etc.' It is difficult to extricate assessment as a separate activity from the general care of the ill person and family.

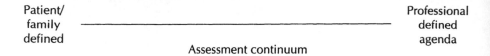

Fig. 2.4   Psychosocial assessment in palliative care

Although palliative care is a very patient-centred activity and good assessment begins with the person's concerns, fears and anxieties, the professional will come with an agenda determined by the *purpose* of the assessment (e.g. for day care, to ease family conflict), the *nature* and *limits* of the *setting* (e.g. hospital support team, specialist HIV/AIDS team) and the professional *role* being performed (e.g. nurse, counsellor).

In some situations one can remain primarily patient/family-led in the entire process of assessment (see Fig. 2.4). However in others, the focus may have to shift, certainly at times, to a more professional-led approach, when what one offers is largely either determined by the resources and policy of the agency or the specific nature of the request for assessment, e.g. patient's mental health, money for bills. This does not negate the need to always be person-centred. The skilled professional will reconcile and integrate these two agendas and find a place on the Assessment Continuum. In practice, the assessment will move up and down the continuum. In any case, personal and cultural factors will always remain important (Geissler, 1994).

The process of assessment will affect and influence the ill person and family. It will provide opportunities to intervene therapeutically. Assessment involves our full range of professional knowledge, skills and values, and locates areas of concern, risk, problems and issues. Assessment likewise identifies potential for change and the ill person/family's resources and strengths on which to build. Assessment involves negotiating with the ill person/family.

Confidentiality

We mention issues of confidentiality in practice from the outset of this book as it is an important area and links with respect for the ill person and his family. It is particularly related to assessment as much new information is being received by the individuals in the team; however, there are, of course, issues concerning confidentiality throughout the period of the person's care.

For all the professionals interviewed, issues of confidentiality were raised. This was evident in concern expressed that as palliative care professionals working in multi-professional teams, we often subscribe to the ethic that information is confidential to the team, not necessarily to be kept by the person who received the information. There was discomfort that so much information was shared openly and not sufficient care taken to be sensitive to discern if it was something appropriate. There was a strong feeling that this could infringe the rights of the client in reducing the control he has over what he divulges or discusses. For many, particularly in the field of work with people with AIDS, but not exclusively, the patient's history or current circumstances can so easily become the focus of curious interest rather than of direct use in clinical involvement.

The question of who should be party to information is complex: should health care assistants and volunteers be expected to share information which the patient has confided in them? Should counsellors working in psychologically painful areas of a person's life be expected to impart information received within a counselling relationship. Should ward or day centre volunteers know the patient's diagnosis or prognosis?

Particularly in a hospital setting, where the ill person may feel stripped of their identity and autonomy, it is essential that patients retain some control of the information about them and with whom it is shared. Therefore, a careful checking process with the patient is advocated strongly. The team's working agreement on confidentiality should be clarified verbally with the patient and also available to them in written form, for example in leaflets describing the service.

Framework for holistic assessment

Holistic assessment involves the total person: body, mind and spirit. Even if one is a 'psychosocial professional', it is essential to work closely with other colleagues whose primary task is to work with the other dimensions.

Body, mind, spirit

In carrying out an assessment in whatever role, one attempts to consider the whole person and their circumstances: *body*, *mind* and *spirit*. The interaction of these three aspects shapes the person and their uniqueness. The 52-year-old man in excruciating pain with terminal cancer, when asked by the palliative care team on their first visit to identify the help he needed most, immediately turned to his wife and said, '*She's* going to be left with all the bills.' Because of the interaction between physical and psychological pain, identifying the social or financial pain on assessment was essential in offering intervention on the ill person's terms.

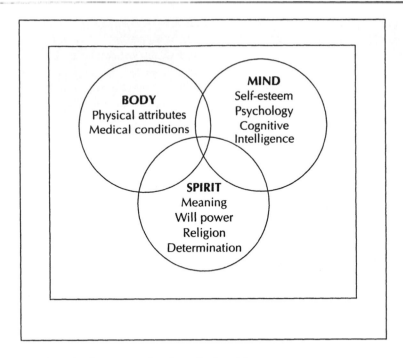

Fig. 2.5   The whole person: body, mind, spirit
The diagram specifically shows the person's attributes of body, mind and spirit as overlapping entities.

The whole person

When making a holistic assessment, i.e. very aware of the whole person, it is essential that we take into account the wide networks of family, community and society. The person never exists in isolation but lives in a context. Even the very isolated, elderly patient living alone and with no relatives is, in part, a product of the attitudes of the local community, legislation, cultural norms and patterns and local health and government policies and procedures.

One needs to take into account three areas of a person's life:

★ Environmental needs
   ● Housing conditions, e.g. adapted or not.
   ● Financial circumstances, e.g. can bills be paid?
   ● Material conditions at home, e.g. sub-standard housing?
   ● Facilities and resources in the neighbourhood, e.g. local libraries.

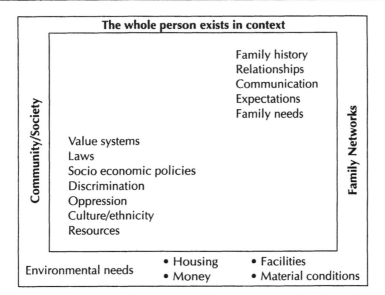

The whole person exists in context

Community/Society

Family Networks

Family history
Relationships
Communication
Expectations
Family needs

Value systems
Laws
Socio economic policies
Discrimination
Oppression
Culture/ethnicity
Resources

Environmental needs

- Housing
- Money

- Facilities
- Material conditions

Fig. 2.6   Framework for holistic assessment

★ Family and networks

- Family history, e.g. previous deaths
- Important relationships and their quality, e.g. who does ill person worry about most?
- Communication patterns, e.g. are they supportive or hostile?
- Expectations of the family/carers, e.g. cultural requirements
- Family needs, e.g. to provide for dependent family members

★ Community and society

- Value systems to which ill person/family is subject, e.g. old people treated with respect
- Laws that permit or ban, e.g. euthanasia
- Discrimination or oppression, e.g. certain groups are disadvantaged and experience unequal opportunities
- Culture and ethnicity, e.g. what are the specific requirements, based on religious or cultural expectations?
- Resources, e.g. social and health care services.

Our work in palliative care is as good as the assessments and reassessments we make. No effective work can be carried out without knowing our consumers. In a field of work that has always valued the uniqueness and individuality of the experience of the patient/family, assessment is the key and a critical starting point to handing back as much control to the person whose body is out of their control.

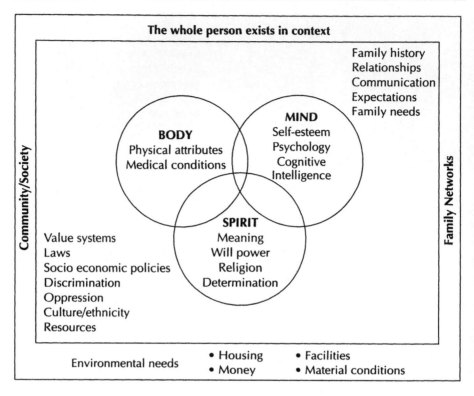

Fig. 2.7   Framework for holistic assessment – the whole person exists in a context

3 Working with families

'Far more people are affected by disease than are infected by it.'
(Anderson, 1995)

The family as the unit of care has long been one of the sacred philosophies of palliative care. How this is translated into the realities of responding to the needs of distressed families, often in crisis, is the content of this chapter. 'The family is far greater than the sum of its membership and the challenge for us is to work with the family group, focusing on its characteristics and interactions rather than on each member in turn' (Gelcer, 1983).

The work described in this chapter is based on the practice of a social worker, a family therapist and a psychologist, all of whom have had extensive experience of working with families in both hospice and palliative care in hospital settings, in homes as well as in a clinical base.

Family histories, myths, roles and relationships are powerful. One experienced practitioner related how she often enquires of a palliative care patient, 'What would your grandmother have said?' (Odier, 1996). For many patients, the wisdom or otherwise of their family members can be quite influential. The question itself leads to insights into the powerful issues with which the patient is struggling.

'Cancer can affect a family in much the same way as it invades the body, causing it to deteriorate if left untreated' (Parkes, 1975). Therefore good practice in palliative care will include good practice in working with the family.

A hospice team working with families: a family-focused approach

Janet Foster, Senior Social Worker, St Luke's Hospice, Sheffield

St Luke's Hospice is a 25-bed hospice with three day units providing 15 places per day and open five days per week. A Macmillan Support Team with six nurses supports patients at home. The bereavement service covers families with links with the hospice or with the hospital-based Macmillan nurses. St Luke's Hospice is situated in Sheffield, a city with half a million population. The hospice is well established and is internationally known and respected. Many leading figures in hospice and palliative care have had working links with St Luke's.

Looking beyond the patient

Janet Foster emphasises the need for the multi-professional team to look beyond the patient to the family – meaning those people important to the ill person. Serious illness affects everyone. Much of Janet's practice describes a strategy for working with families in an in-patient unit and day centre, although not exclusively, as the ill person moves between in-patient care, day care and home care.

Fifteen years' experience in the palliative care field has given Janet broad exposure to the many pressures, anxieties and fears families face when confronted with serious illness. Examples include the pressures on individual members 'to keep feelings to themselves and to maintain a brave face' and a cheerful exterior to avoid upsetting each other; difference in levels of understanding about the illness and expectations; practical adjustments and role changes in how the family operates; and worries about the future, living with uncertainty and anxieties about what will happen.

The ill person and his family influence each other in the way they respond to and cope with illness. Getting to really know the family is, therefore, an essential part of the overall assessment of the ill person.

The multi-professional team recognises the need for family-focused work from initial referral through to bereavement. When a nurse compiles the records of a new patient, the family tree and other significant information about family, friends and carers are included under the heading 'Family and Support Network'.

The hospice brochure, given to the ill person and family, includes a pull-out section for families. The nurse undertaking admission procedures will routinely see family members and include them in the whole process. Part of this process is a two-way flow of information between hospice staff and family about the care of the ill person, main concerns at that stage and practical arrangements in the hospice.

When the doctor first meets the ill person, he or she will meet the relative, if available. However, the nursing team leader will automatically try and see the relative or main carer.

The social worker in the team is particularly identified with specialist family support. He or she will screen all referral forms to identify clues that might indicate if additional involvement is needed, e.g. 'the patient is also caring for a daughter with a disability'; 'a very recent diagnosis and the family is very distressed'; 'longstanding marital difficulties'. It is important not to make assumptions. Subjective comments, e.g. 'difficult families' or 'aggressive wife' may have been made without any indication of what led to the behaviour. These kind of descriptions always need unravelling in order to get behind the labels.

The social worker's daily contact with the team leader updates information on newly admitted patients and needs. The ongoing 'screening' of patients and working with the nurse's knowledge of the family identifies gaps and need for intervention. If a relative has not manifested, the social worker will take the initiative to make telephone contact: 'We've been thinking of you and wondering how you are.'

The multi-professional team

Weekly multi-professional team meetings discuss all 25 patients with the doctors, nurses, social workers as well as the chaplain, art therapist and physiotherapist adding their observations.

A standard question, 'how's the family?', allows some reflection on needs, levels of distress and anxieties about the future among the family members, to be shared. Different perceptions are integrated and the need to involve other specialists or agencies identified. For example, the aromatherapist, while helping patients relax, hears a great deal about their family concerns. These are shared with the wider team within the context of the team policy on confidentiality.

Part of the success in identifying family needs and working with the family's resources, is the experience of the multi-professional team working together as a 'family'. The commonality of experience, history and language, while respecting different perceptions, forms a structure and context to discuss family issues. The team cannot begin agreeing a new set of working concepts and mores for each new family; they need some common ground. Yet they recognise the uniqueness of each family and the importance of meeting the family on *their* terms.

A key relationship and source of information is the nursing team who get to know the families well. The team leader does not wait for the families to approach them; she initiates contact with the family, especially as the ill person's condition changes and medication alters.

Teams also change in composition, as staff leave and are replaced. The family-focused approach has to be persistently maintained within the team which has to repeatedly redefine its ethos and task. This involves training and careful joint discussion of observations about a family among members of the team.

Family assessment enquires:

- Who are the significant people?
- Are there any specific requirements concerning their language, culture, diet, religion?
- Are their relationships close or distant, longstanding or recently formed?
- How easy or difficult is it for the family to talk to each other?
- How do they communicate, e.g. is news passed on, do they visit together or separately, do they seek out or avoid staff?
- Who might be particularly vulnerable?
- Is anyone being left out?
- Have there been any recent deaths or other major life changes?
- What role did the patient have within the family, e.g. carer? Who is filling that role now and what gap is left?
- Has the patient's personality changed since the illness?
- Are there any immediate needs or concerns, e.g. help with taxi fares, or additional care for someone at home?
- What needs might there be in the future?

Preparing families

Much of the work with families forms a continuing preparation for the next stage of the illness and for death. Information and support are key tools.

From first contact a message is given that the hospice or palliative care team is interested in the family. This is often reinforced by the resources available: an additional bed for relatives to stay if necessary, open visiting, playroom/toys and games for children, the extension of basic hospitality to friends and family, the provision of leaflets with general information projecting the message 'you are important.'

The multi-professional team will decide who will take the family a step further, e.g. if it is largely more medical information that is required, it may be the doctor, if it involves working with conflictual relationships, it may be the social worker but not necessarily. Increasingly, it may involve a joint interview.

The hospice/palliative care unit supports families by:

- Making the unit a welcoming place
- Providing a section in the brochure for families
- Having open visiting
- Inviting relatives to stay overnight, if necessary
- Allowing family to be involved in the care, if they wish
- Involving a member of the team for additional support

- Housing a small sitting room for families
- Recording specific requirements respecting ethnicity.

What is our role as practitioners with families?

- To provide a safe environment, either at home or in the unit
- Sometimes neutral ground is more appropriate, particularly when there is family conflict
- To make short, clear statements, introductions, why we are meeting, areas to talk about, etc.
- To observe family interaction: body language, use of touch, how they handle distress and tears
- To listen and give everyone the opportunity to talk and share concerns ask questions, etc.
- To acknowledge their difficulties and dilemmas
- To be honest about *our* uncertainties, about the way the illness will progress
- To affirm their contribution and emphasise the positives
- To make it acceptable to talk about sensitive areas, e.g. angry feelings towards each other, resentment towards the ill person, relief at the death
- To agree on a plan. This may be very short term or limited but it is important that everyone is clear about contact from the team.

Some observations and practice issues in working with families:

- We must remember that families are anxious and may require reassurance
- Mention that it is standard practice that we meet the family of a patient
- Large families are not necessarily close families
- We must not be intrusive or overwhelm families. Sensitive timing is important
- The team needs to have a clear plan to avoid giving mixed messages.
- Families need to retain control
- We are only there to help them to sort things out for themselves, not take over
- We may have met this situation many times before but it is likely to be the first time for them. We need to allow ample time to go over issues and to repeat information
- We are there for everyone in the family – try to avoid taking sides
- We need to recognise the value of short-term work – one meeting may be sufficient.

Identifying families at risk

Significant factors which are thought to pre-dispose a family to emotional 'risk' include:

- Recent diagnosis of advanced illness; family very shocked by the diagnosis
- Expressed anger about delays in diagnosis or aspects of treatment
- Close dependent relationship with the ill person
- Children or adolescent in the family
- Other pressures and demands, e.g. caring for elderly parents
- Carer very isolated with very little support
- Previous or current mental health problem
- Previous losses, especially if recent
- Practical difficulties such as finance, housing and employment
- Not realistic about the patient's prognosis
- Evidence of drug/alcohol dependency
- Conflict/tensions within the family
- Estranged family members
- Family members who might be excluded, e.g. people with learning disabilities
- History of abuse, trauma or a 'disorganised' family.

A systemic approach to working with families

Margi Abeles, Family Therapist

Margi Abeles is a hospital staff counsellor and freelance family therapist, working with individuals, couples and families. She specialises in work with families facing death and bereavement. For many years she worked as a medical social worker and a social worker in a hospice home care, in-patient and day unit. She was also a member of the Jewish bereavement counselling service.

A family, as with a group, is more than the sum of its parts, as has been mentioned. It has a life of its own which is tested by the crisis of diagnosis, treatment, terminal illness, death and bereavement. With strong emotions in confronting the inevitability of death, we are often left 'managing the unmanageable', with families. In palliative care we attempt 'to create a safe space for the family to talk about difficult issues' (Margi Abeles). This section looks at what using systems and family therapy principles and practices mean when applied to hospice and palliative care.

Families as systems

In families, what one person does affects another. Within a system, one part is dependent on another to ensure the whole works smoothly. Families develop unwritten rules and ways of behaving to help the members function well. These mechanisms offer the family unit stability and predictability. The rules help people know how to act. The family becomes a living organism in its own right. Members take on roles and responsibilities and ways of dealing with problems, maintaining the family's 'equilibrium' and 'homeostatis' despite daily upheavals. In simple terms, each family member knows his/her own role and task and the family works as an integrated team for much of the time: *the family system*. Some families display extreme behaviour.

According to Carter and McGoldrick (1988), a family may be thought of as the entire emotional system of three or four generations of people who have a strong emotional involvement that exists through time. Thus, the family may include persons both living and deceased. Family patterns, rules, myths and secrets originating in the past may be powerfully present in the current emotional functioning of the family. Consequently, family history may be as important as the current family composition. Behaviour which seems odd may make sense when placed in historical context and the influence of the family's chronology is understood.

Systemic thinking helps us consider the family and the effect of wider systems and influences on the ill person and his world, e.g. the hospital, the primary care team, the multi-professional team in the specialist unit. It recognises the different contexts in which the ill person lives: work, religious group, neighbourhood, and how they react and interact with the ill person. It is based on the premise that an individual view is limited in its usefulness. A systemic approach thinks of the ill person in all his significant relationships and networks and in the wider context of society. We cannot understand the whole while looking at the individual parts. The meaning of behaviour has to be understood in context.

Family therapy

Family therapy is based on the idea that the behaviour of individuals and families is influenced and maintained by the ways other individuals and systems interact with them. The wife who does not talk about the prognosis is not on her own: her husband does not ask or hear either. They 'hold' each other in the situation of denial. In systems thinking, any movement in one part of the system or family, will have a corresponding movement in another part – almost a see-saw effect.

If behaviour is dependent on context, we have to go away from seeing it as 'just in the person'. For example, consider a 'miserable' person. 'Misery' may not be in that person intrinsically but 'this is a person who shows misery in that particular context.'

Families and palliative care

In palliative care, we employ thinking and skills from the field of family therapy, rather than using 'pure' family therapy, although there are, of course, families who require just that.

Practice example

Jim, 25, is a single man living at home with his parents. There was poor communication between Jim and his parents since he disclosed his AIDS diagnosis. An only child, Jim had lived away from home since he was 17. Jim's GP had contacted the hospice requesting a respite care bed urgently as Jim's parents were having great difficulty nursing him at home. Jim's mother had also directly contacted the hospice.

With the crisis of the diagnosis of life-threatening or terminal illness and death, the family system is thrown *off-balance*, coping with a situation with which it has probably never previously dealt and for which it has to evolve some new rules.

Perceiving the picture of the family in terms of the system enables us to organise and make sense of the sometimes quite complex, confusing and conflicting phenomena with which we are presented, in terms of relationships, attitudes and past experience. In palliative care, there is always a proportion of families who are particularly angry, in conflict, rejecting us and what is being offered. We begin to see the family, not so much as the individuals that are its members, but more as the interactions between them, their patterns of relating, their history, 'games' and roles. The *interconnectedness*, rather than the individuals, is the focus of work. 'Families are viewed as interrelated, interdependent, interacting complex organisms, constantly influencing and being influenced by their environment' (Hall and Kirschling, 1990).

Employing a systemic approach in working with families in the palliative care setting can result in a variety of methods and techniques. However, what is crucial is that a systemic approach shapes the thinking and understanding around families and how they function. Systems thinking opens up different explanations into the behaviour of the family members which widens choice as compared with individual-focused models and theories (Smith, 1990; Smith and Regnard, 1993).

The systems and family therapy practice perspective can be useful in palliative care whether one is directly working with an individual ill person or carer, multi-professional team or colleague from another agency.

Systems thinking at various stages of intervention

The referral

Referrals often result in pressure of work on top of a full workload. New patients bring a new set of stories, often emotive and horrific. Stop. Think. Get a team response. Plan. There is frequently pressure to act quickly.

The information recorded at the point of referral may say more about the needs of the person referring than the actual situation of the ill person. The ill person is at the centre of a pattern of interlocking relationships and his experience is determined by them. We cannot think of the ill person in isolation from their partners, children, parents, friends, etc. It is a helpful aid if the referral form has space for a genogram ('family tree' or 'relationship tree') which gives a pictorial view of the family.

It is essential that the team pause for a moment to speculate around the referral: who is referring? what is it *they* are anxious about? what is the pressure on them? We need to explore different explanations for what is happening.

It is important to underline the difference between *reacting* and *responding* to the newly referred situation. *Reacting* can be very immediate, taking action about demands, requests and pressure to do something urgently. It relieves one's own anxieties. *Responding* requires more discernment of needs and the best way of meeting these. It requires some pause for thought and is a way of managing anxiety in the team, just when the glaring need is huge and the individual professional or team is being made to feel incompetent, unless some intervention is made immediately.

The result of the referral on Jim was a realisation that little of Jim's voice was being heard and that there was a strong concern from his GP. Rather than immediately offering a bed, the team decided that the medical director should talk to the GP about what exactly lay behind his concern and that the social worker should speak to Jim and his family. It transpired that the GP was a friend of Jim's parents and that work on communication within the family reduced the tension in caring for Jim.

There is more than one explanation for what is going on in a family. Being able to step back and to consider the dynamics is part of the process of working with families.

Labelling and assumptions

Families are referred with various labels, e.g. 'difficult', 'anxious', 'Jewish', 'Asian'. Using systemic thinking, one would make a hypothesis to understand what the interrelationships are and be prepared to test this out with the ill person and family.

Planning the first visit or interview

Never make the assumption that you, as a professional, know best who should be there. If possible, find out from the ill person who they would like to be present. The response may give you a clue to the openness of the family. If possible, try to meet the ill person together with those closest to him.

The first family meeting will provide an opportunity: to explore the nature of the crisis of the illness and what it means to the family; to begin to identify the strengths and resources which the family has, and to enable the members to draw on the support of their relationships. The early meetings will also establish a foundation of trust with the professionals, communication and co-operation.

Contract

Normalise the opportunity to talk together with the family. For example, we sometimes say, 'As a team, we like to have a chance to meet the family.' Acknowledge the invitation, not the prescription. We need to engage family members in a way that is unthreatening.

A contract or agreement, however simple, must be made as to why you are there and how you are going to work together. The purpose of the visit or interview needs to be made explicit, even if the aims are modest: 'I wanted to introduce myself today, so that you would know who you were speaking to if you had any worries.' A contract avoids the misunderstandings: when someone might be thinking you are there for one purpose (e.g. providing financial support) whilst you have prioritised another area (e.g. talking about death and dying).

Equally you need to allow the family to be attentive to areas they do not wish to discuss by saying something like, 'Stop us when we're talking about things you'd rather not discuss.' This builds in safety and control. Bearing in mind that in palliative care much contact is very short term, subsequent meetings can draw on these foundations.

Family meetings

We often comment to families, 'illness affects everyone in the family', not only to engage them but to demonstrate that understanding their individual experiences are connected, e.g. *he* does not take the morphine because *she* gets upset. Even children can appreciate that 'illness is like throwing a pebble in the sea; it causes many ripples.' Indeed, it is not uncommon for the youngest members of the family to begin to reveal the family dynamics.

The use of generalisation can be effective in initiating family meetings as with individual interviews: 'many families tell us that they experience ... what is it like for you?' or, for example, 'from our experience of listening to many families in your situation ... we find that children who have a chance to talk openly before can have an easier time afterwards.' This projects the safety of knowing that others share the experience but does not deny the unique quality of this particular experience.

Family meetings are often held with several members or a few. Two colleagues working together, e.g. doctor and social worker or nurse and psychologist, can be effective, as issues can become very weighty and mutual support and two sets of observations are beneficial. Two different professionals can cover different aspects of the illness between them but can also take contrasting roles during the family meeting, for example, one active interviewer and the other the active observer. The way the two communicate with each other can demonstrate the importance of negotiating together and that differing and tentative views can be held by the professionals.

Neutrality

Neutrality is a factor in family therapy. When you are with a family, you would like to be perceived as being allied to all and none of the family members at the same time. This sometimes needs saying directly to the family, particularly when there is clear conflict. Move the conversation around so that everyone can be included. Be aware of your own ideas and of how these can be imposed on others. We exercise authority and power and we need to be sensitive to the fact that as professionals, and from an official service, we can be at risk of abusing it. Cultural issues have also to be acknowledged, e.g. the possible implications of a woman talking to an Asian man.

If we begin to get over-involved or 'sucked into' a situation, we limit our usefulness, e.g. a nurse very close to the wife may inadvertently make the husband feel left out. Monroe (1993a) warns: 'If the family find balance only with and in your presence, you have become part of the problem rather than helping them find an answer.'

Genograms/family trees/relationship trees

Genograms, also known as family or relationship trees, are assessment tools providing valuable information on previous losses, illnesses and deaths as well as supportive relationships. The genogram provides opportunity to discuss the family's fears, concerns and hopes (McGoldrick and Gerson, 1985). Drawing the family tree with the family or individual provides rich opportunities to talk and to grieve. Children will often be the most comfortable in 'mentioning the unmentionables' (Smith and Pennells, 1995).

Working in the 'here and now'

Watching and using what is going on in the room in front of you is the essence of working systemically: communication patterns, seating positions, what happens when something particular is mentioned. All these phenomena can be commented on and discussed to enable the family to behave in a different way. For example, 'I notice when Mum begins to cry, Jim talks about getting better.' The *pattern* and *process* of relating together is as much the focus of work as listening to the *content* of what is being said.

Being curious

It is important to put away assumptions and enquire about what this particular family wants and does things. Exploration is part of the work. 'She's depressed', says the carer. Find out the meaning of that depression to the individual and to the family. Help the family define the problem or phenomena with which they are contending: 'What is the most difficult or worrying aspect that you are having to cope with?' 'Who is most affected by mother's illness?' 'Of the many difficulties you have mentioned, which do you find most ...?' 'What would have to happen to make a difference?'

Positive reframing

This strategy tries to change a view and, therefore, behaviour, e.g. the 13-year-old boy whose father is dying and who is being aggressive around the house may be said to be 'showing his grief'.

Positive reframing provides an alternative to a negative view, e.g. the 'how well you are coping with an impossible situation' or 'I admire the way you wish to remain in control' to a patient who has rejected all offers of help. The positive connotation must contain some element of truth.

The multi-professional team

As a team we are a system and we have an effect on the family. For example, it is easy for some members of the team to get split off as 'special' or to come into competition with their colleagues. Care is also required to avoid aspects of team communication, conflict and scapegoating being taken into direct work with families, for example a difficult relationship between doctor and nurse that might be acted out in front of the family.

Supervision

In order to keep direction, good supervision from an appropriate professional with experience in supervision in family work is essential, since we are also part of the system; we need time to talk about how working with families affects us.

Working with children when a family death is expected

Julie Stokes, Consultant Clinical Psychologist at the Gloucester Royal Hospital Palliative Care Team and Programme Director of Winston's Wish

> 'We live in a culture that prefers children to be seen, but not sad.'
> (Julie Stokes)

This section will focus particularly on work with families prior to the death occurring, especially where there are children involved. Julie works as part of the palliative care service, a multi-professional support team, the team which first identified the need for a child bereavement service. As a result, Julie pioneered Winston's Wish, a grief support programme for children aged six to fourteen years old, following the death of someone important in their lives. The Winston's Wish team is a multi-professional team involving people from education, health and social services backgrounds. They are supported by 35 trained volunteers.

Winston's Wish attempts to respond to the individual needs of bereaved children and their families and has a number of aims:

- To organise a service which can offer an intervention to *all* children bereaved of an immediate family member, with the intention of reducing the risk of psychological problems in later life

- To increase a child's knowledge and understanding of death
- To increase a child's awareness and understanding of the grieving process
- To promote open communication with the family
- To respond to the individual needs of each child and its family by enabling them to continue their lives in a meaningful way.

Winston's Wish provides a variety of services but for most families their first involvement will be attending Camp Winston, a residential weekend for children and a non-residential group for parents (Stokes and Crossley, 1995).

Process issues for practitioners in working with families

Practice example

Sue, 34, is married to Pete, 38, and has three children, all girls, aged seven, eight and eleven years old. Sue is diagnosed as having AIDS and her husband is HIV positive as is their youngest daughter.

Much of the work with families is focused on *empowering* parents and carers to communicate with their children. This can happen at an early stage or even the day before the death occurs. Although, in general, one subscribes to the principle of 'never giving advice', this is perhaps an area of work where education and information are invaluable for parents, e.g. highlighting children's common reactions to bad news. Many parents have found it useful to know that their children might respond by being very matter of fact, asking, 'what's for tea?' after being told that their Dad is going to die. Also it is important that as professionals we do not allow families to feel they are failing: 'There are no right answers, just a willingness to do your best – being a "good enough" parent is all any of us can hope to achieve.'

In working alongside a family when someone is expected to die, there are a number of key steps within the process.

Step 1   Where and when do you meet the parents?

Organise a meeting with the parents in a venue which enhances their *control*, for example, at home at a suitable time when the parents can talk freely and express their emotions.

Where possible, involve the referrer. In Sue's case, the AIDS coordinator who made the referral will be continuing to work with the family and it is therefore important that he discusses his concerns and hopes regarding your intervention. Clearly the presence of the referrer depends on the relationship and wishes of the family. In Sue's situation, the family trusted the AIDS coordinator and the acceptance and continuity of the service was promoted by his presence at the first meeting.

Step 2   Helping parents to introduce you to the children

Try to help the *parents* to work out a way of explaining to the children who you are and why you are spending time with the family: 'How are you going to explain to ... why I'm here?' This planning conversation with the parents will effectively become part of the intervention as it forces parents to confront the reality and adapt to a potential death within the family. In addition, the children need to know that their parents approve of you and are comfortable about the situation.

Spend time getting to know the children and what is important to them, e.g. school, best friends, how family life has changed. You need to relax and engage the family by talking about 'normal' family life. Try and elicit funny family stories, so that you and the family remind themselves of life outside cancer, AIDS, etc.

Step 3   Present options to the family

Give the family options of how you could work, e.g. see the child individually, see siblings together, work with the family as a whole, see each parent separately or as a couple, etc. Explain to the children where and when they will be seen. Perhaps give them some simple 'homework' (nothing threatening) that they can bring to your next meeting. Children often feel comfortable bringing toys, photos or other objects that help facilitate a discussion. Recently I saw some children whose sister had died – the children decided to bring bags of toys that had belonged to their sister.

Be aware that with pre-death work in palliative care, you often do not have the opportunity to work in a long-term and planned way. With most families, you may only have a chance of meeting them once or twice. Similarly in terms of workload, you may only be able to undertake extensive work with one or two families. Thus the completion of lengthy memory books, parents writing letters for the surviving children, etc. may not be possible for many families.

The timing of an intervention with families is not only determined by ill health, but by the fact that it takes a while for the family to acknowledge the diagnosis and prognosis.

Step 4   Working with the family system

As you meet with various family members you need to try to understand how each person contributes to the family system. Different people will have different roles and coping strategies that may be seen as 'helpful' or 'unhelpful' in the eyes of the other family members. For example, Sue perceived her middle daughter's tantrums and repeated school refusal as an indication of the fact that she was the one who really cared and thus responded to her behaviour positively, particularly when the daughter remained at home during the day. Pete, however, felt that this difficult behaviour was attention-seeking and highly inappropriate given the family situation. Acknowledgement that the child's behaviour could be interpreted in different ways led to a constructive discussion about managing the behaviour. Pete was able to ask his daughter if the fact that she took a mirror to her mother's face at night indicated her grave concern for mother. The daughter was able to acknowledge that she was very worried about her mother dying suddenly and needed to check her breath in the mirror.

You always need to be aware of trying to maintain a neutral position in the family system. When families are feeling vulnerable, and when communication can be so difficult, it may feel flattering to be taken into the confidence of one person, e.g. mother. However, how will her partner feel if he thinks she is able to confide in you and not in him? This may be particularly hurtful when time is limited for the couple. Pre-death work can be extremely demanding and there is often a tendency to go for easier options, i.e. colluding more than we would in less emotionally-charged situations. Even experienced practitioners can be drawn into 'changing' usual patterns of professional behaviour and become over-involved. Palliative care calls on the individual professional to make a personal and human response whilst working in a team context. In a speciality that emphasises the uniqueness of the experience, we can easily take a leap over the helping relationship boundary in our attempt to 'feel with the client'. Regular professional supervision is essential.

Acknowledge to yourself that your contract as a palliative care practitioner is not only to communicate directly with the family but to work with other professionals in order to ease the way *they* communicate with the family or carry out their task. Thus you may find yourself needing to be sensitive to colleagues' anxieties and concerns. A conversation with a colleague in front of children is sometimes a useful strategy for opening up issues and modelling appropriate behaviour. For example, you may start up a conversation with a GP in front of a child: 'This is John and he was wondering about his Dad and what sort of medicine you would be giving him so that his Dad is comfortable? ... John also wanted you to know that he wants to be kept in the picture – particularly when you think his Dad is about to die.'

On one occasion, when Sue's daughters appeared on the ward to see their mother who had gone into a coma, the nurses were clearly fearful as to how they would handle the situation. The nurses were put at their ease when we said, 'The children know that they probably cannot talk to their mum today but we've brought some bags of clay to make something, so if mum wakes up she'll know the girls have been.' This engaged the nurses who relaxed and immediately involved themselves in helping the children make their clay models.

Step 5   After the death

Eventually, when the patient has died, it is crucial that the family understand your continuing role. Ideally this should be negotiated when the patient is alive so they can feel comfortable about the ongoing support the family will receive after the death.

We need to be clear with families what we can or cannot offer. It can be difficult to talk about withdrawing from a family having shared the intensity of a pre-death experience. However, we need to be realistic about how much contact we can have. This also prepares the way for acceptance of our colleagues who will undertake bereavement work.

Step 6   Endings

Plan your departure from the family carefully. You have become part of the family system and the members need to prepare for your disconnection just as they have done when their relative was ill and died.

Try to arrange supervision for yourself so you can understand what emotional connections you have developed with this family. Without supervision, you may find yourself giving unrealistic commitments, for example, it would not be helpful for Sue to see Julie as a surrogate mother. There is sometimes a hidden drive by the family to encourage you to form overtly close relationships. Others may view you with potential to 'make things better'. Such expectations are unrealistic and families need to space to grieve.

Being alongside a family and doing pre-death work is both demanding and a privilege. There are no set right and wrong ways to respond. However, it does help everyone if you feel confident with your role and not overwhelmed by the tragic circumstances facing the family.

Some practice ideas used

Memory boxes

As the name states, the 'memory box' gives a dying or surviving relative a chance to create a collection of special mementoes, writings or paintings to capture some memories. One of the best-known boxes has been produced by Barnardos. The 'Memory Store' aims to help parents whose children face separation from them to gather and store the information and memories which will be so important in their children's future (Neville, 1995).

The Memory Store is a brightly coloured box. Inside are drawers where the special and important memories of family life and childhood can be stored. It is possible to include a video of family celebrations, birthdays, holidays. Notes on 'a day in the life of' the family, favourite foods and activities can be included as well as objects and souvenirs valued by the parent. The Memory Store has a memory book with sheets which help parents write down facts about their own and their children's lives.

Nowadays we are even more conscious of the value of biography, stories and memories as part of the process of grieving (Walter, 1996). A memory box helps the child piece together the story of the deceased relative and take them into their lives and into the future.

Obviously the creation of the memory box by the ill parent can be extremely painful. The timing and pacing for what seems right to them is, of course, essential. However, the memory box has potential to give not only information about the past in terms of the family history but also details of the deceased parent's life as a child.

A man aged 30 whose wife had become pregnant, and whose mother had died after a long illness when he was aged eight, realised he never knew his birth weight. In itself, this may not be of overwhelming importance but it exemplifies the absence of a store of family life stories from the past.

Part of the agenda in doing this work is being very conscious of *who* the client is. In working with Sue's youngest daughter, then aged seven, Julie was conscious that she would also have needs as a 17-year-old teenager, and then again at 27, perhaps with children of her own. At all these stages she would benefit from information and tangible memories in the box to assist her in piecing together the story of her past, when other memories might have faded. Thus part of our work sometimes involves taking the parent into their child's future, to 'second-guess' what they imagine may be helpful in keeping the memory of themselves 'alive'. As one child said, 'I want to be able to say "hello" to my Mum not "goodbye" – alive or dead.' The memory box also has the potential to open up conversations and give opportunities for children to recount their stories of life before their relative died.

Sue included in the memory box for her children: photos, jewellery, little teddy bears and a video of her watching her children in the school Christmas play.

A grandfather whose 40-year-old daughter was dying, found her imminent death extremely painful to discuss openly. He 'spoke' his feelings by carefully making some beautiful memory boxes for the grandchildren. The needs of grandparents are quite often neglected and this practical task helped him enormously. It is beneficial to give the parent or grandparent a 'menu' of different media they can use in making the memory box and it is important not to create a situation in which they feel guilty if they do not manage to do a conventional memory box.

Anger wall

Anger can be a key emotion for families. It is often difficult to express verbally and creative alternatives can be useful.

There is always something people are angry about. The anger wall is a trigger in acknowledging angry feelings and provides a safe outlet for each family member's own specific disappointments and expressions of anger. Providing an opportunity to throw 'clay bombs' at named targets on a wall, can only be done in certain environments.

Utilising an 'anger wall' depends on the health of the palliative care patient. At the time the anger wall was used with Sue's family, she was already very weak and in a wheelchair. The exercise was adapted to allow Sue to participate. For example, it surprised everyone how outraged Dad was at one particular doctor. Similarly Mum was able to express her anger at leaving the family and it was important for the children to hear that. Although she herself was too weak to throw, she in turn participated by giving the children the clay bombs to throw on her behalf.

Sue then suggested that the anger be made more constructive and the clay fashioned into different animals. She further participated by choosing which animal she felt appropriate. For example, she chose a chimpanzee for her husband who kept a happy face and cheered everyone up. She wanted him to know that that was something she valued. She chose a butterfly for one of the girls whom she felt was quite delicate and so on. The children then made these animals out of the clay and they were kept safely in their memory boxes. After Sue had died the children then had a 'story' to tell that helped them stay 'connected' to Mum.

Trying to be imaginative and yet using material which would naturally mean something for a particular family with whom you are working, is a challenge and should be carefully negotiated so that the activity fits the family style.

Letters

These are sometimes written by a dying parent to a child with the intention of them being opened at some time in the future, e.g. going to university, wedding day. The use of letters should be approached with caution as they can leave the recipient with a strong feeling that they have a set of instructions which should be obeyed in deference to the deceased. A letter can be quite prescriptive in its contents and contain unrealistic expectations. Thus what if the son or daughter decides not to marry? A general letter, for example, for a child when adult, is safer.

The palliative care team negotiated time off school for a teenager whose mother was expected to die shortly. The daughter 'interviewed' her mother about various aspects of her life and created a booklet to look back on. The daughter was able to clarify clouded areas, e.g. 'What do you mean, I'll work with children? What happens if I don't?' This led to a more meaningful interchange.

These practice ideas are clearly a *means* to an *end*. The key aims which they have in common are:

- to find a comfortable vehicle to involve children. (Many teachers, parents and other carers are in major discomfort discussing death and bereavement.)
- to communicate to children, 'Yes, you are very important in all this; someone crucial in your life is about to die and you are valued.'
- to show adults that children are robust and that they can be positively involved in their parent's palliative care.
- to lessen complications in bereavement.

The key times of intervention with families facing terminal illness and bereavement are:

- diagnosis
- understanding the diagnosis and treatments
- relationships with the medical team
- the deteriorating body
- medical procedures
- hospitalisation
- relapse
- cessation of treatment
- terminal phase
- death
- funeral
- bereavement.

Conclusion

When a couple are expecting a baby, we accept the need to prepare them by giving information, discussing anxieties, answering questions and providing ante-natal classes. This continues throughout the pregnancy and afterwards and promotes the parents' sense of control and self-esteem. Such preparation helps families adapt to the changing family dynamics resulting from a new baby. So why do we respond so negatively when a family needs to adapt to a potential death? Surely it is not acceptable to ignore family needs simply because one life event is perceived as a happy one (birth) and the other is sad (death)?

Psychological well-being, the enhancement of self-esteem and positive family communication is crucial at a time when life is so fragmented. Research has shown that negative experiences can live with children for the rest of their lives (Black, 1994). Often it is the way a death is handled that complicates a bereavement as opposed to the death *per se*. The skill is not just giving information but in working out what information adults and children want (Stokes, Wyer and Crossley, 1997).

We live in a culture that prefers children to be seen but not sad. Having an open conversation with a child does *not* require elaborate training. However, it does require a willingness to be alongside children when they are both happy and sad, regardless of what feelings it generates in ourselves.

Overview of working with families

The practices described in this chapter have highlighted the significance of the family and caring networks as a vehicle for change. The practitioner cannot replace the family but can respect and promote their capacity for change. With families with children, our role is, in many ways, to show that children can be sad and yet survive.

The family has a continuity: a past and a future. We, as practitioners, usually see a snapshot of the family during a period of crisis and growth. Families have the potential to emerge strengthened from the crisis. As practitioners we help the family to create positive memories of the period of illness, death and bereavement, and to maximise this potential, so that out of the crisis, the family can emerge a different but safe place for its members. The actual death is always a shock, even when talked about very openly. You can never prepare a family enough.

Resources

Traumatic Stress Clinic 73 Charlotte Street, London W1P 1LB. Tel: 0171 436 9000 Fax 0171 436 8800 A national referral centre for adults, children and families

Barnardo's Memory Store Barnardo's Trading Estate, Paycocke Road, Basildon, Essex, SS14 3DR. Tel: 01268 520224

'All About Me' Board Game also from Barnardo's. A board game using a simple snakes and ladders-style board. Players respond to questions in a pack of cards which encourages exchange between practitioner and child

'The Grief Game' (1996), Jessica Kingsley, 116 Pentonville Road, London N1 9JB. Tel: 0171 833 2307

Lifegames is a series of therapeutic board games for children and adolescents, devised to facilitate the understanding and disclosure of the complex feelings experienced

4 Working with groups

'It seemed like a better alternative to painting Easter Eggs ...'
(A member's comment on his motivation for attending a group for
terminally ill people.)

We all spend our lives in groups of one form or another, for example our family and friendship networks. Learning to socialise is a very basic part of human development. Small children are sent to playgroups and nurseries to encourage them to socialise and share and the majority of us spend our education and working lives in groups of some sort. Very ill or bereaved adults and children often feel excluded from the groups to which they had previously belonged. They fear that talking about their feelings may cause embarrassment, and the reaction when they do often confirms their suspicions. The relevance of group work in palliative care is clear. Groups can help promote people to feel less lonely and isolated; they offer opportunities for mutual support and problem solving, a safe place to express feelings and ideas, feedback on behaviour and improved self-esteem through the opportunity to give support as well as to receive it (Yalom, 1995). Bottomley's review on the efficacy of cancer support groups concludes that they 'offer the potential for cost-effective help to cancer patients' (Bottomley, 1997). A randomised controlled trial by Spiegel et al. (1989) even suggested that participation in support groups might prolong the survival of individuals with cancer.

Groups also offer particularly potent opportunities to return power and control to the members rather than the 'professional leaders'. Yet, despite its obvious relevance to palliative care, group work has been used less often than might be expected. The reason for this may be related to resource issues, but the more significant reason appears to be the suspicion and anxiety with which group work is regarded both by professional staff, relatives and friends of potential group members, and of course, group members themselves.

Professionals and carers often seem to fear that distress may be contagious and that in the group setting it may get out of control or make the group members' general behaviour more difficult to manage, leading to a sort of 'don't rock the boat' mentality. There are also anxieties about what may be revealed in the group about other members of the network, particularly if this comment may be negative. In addition, potential group members themselves may never have attended something that identifies itself as a formal group and may worry about safety and about exposure (Sheldon, 1997). In a group for terminally ill people at St Christopher's Hospice one person hoped it was not going to be a 'psycho thingy' and another described bringing the newspaper to his first meeting so he could hide behind it if things got too unbearable. He commented: 'When you are unwell you lose your confidence too.' Group leaders may feel that group work is daunting, something beyond their time, resources or experience. Overcoming the above obstacles may be the most significant factors in a group's success or failure. However all the usual issues surrounding planning for group work will need careful consideration.

This chapter will continue with an outline of the key planning issues. It will then look in detail at the organisation and content of three different groups in order to illustrate specific responses to the points of principle and to examine what actually happens to promote good practice. The groups have been chosen to reflect contrasting methods: ongoing open membership group work, a single-session, highly focused group and a long-term closed group.

Group structure

The purpose of the group – identifying need

Why run a group at all? What are its objectives? An example might be that of single-session open bereavement groups held monthly at St Christopher's Hospice where the objectives are to:

- Normalise feelings to reassure and to help people realise they are not alone
- Facilitate expression of a range of feelings
- Encourage individuals to acknowledge their grief in some way
- Ensure that each individual is heard.

Policy considerations

Who should be included in discussions about the group at this early stage, e.g. team, colleagues, other professionals involved with potential group members?

Group method

The type of group will need to be considered. Dwivedi (1993) makes a useful distinction between experiential and psycho-educational groups. In the latter the workers determine most of the agenda and activity by leading discussions and perhaps using exercises. In an experiential group the therapeutic aspects of the situation that each group member creates within the group are skilfully harnessed by the facilitators.

Group boundaries

The group must set a few ground rules:

- How long will it run for?
- What will the length of each meeting be?
- Will there be a fixed membership or can new members join after the group has been formed?
- What will the frequency of meetings be?

Ongoing and unstructured groups often offer participants the opportunity to attend when they want and are able to. There are also more roles available to participants, for example, they can become mentors or assistants in the running of the group. Disadvantages often cluster around the difficulties of encouraging people to leave. Some hospices have found that open bereavement support meetings can become places where the newly bereaved find it difficult to express distressed and powerful feelings because the bulk of the membership have moved on to more social objectives. Goal setting can help with the problem of termination – an agreement for example, that each member attends for a year from their own start date. Structured, closed-end groups provide an opportunity to define membership and to give participants the sense of closure and accomplishment. The agenda can be planned to meet specific needs and group leaders can plan for a specific time commitment. Disadvantages can be the need to insist on regular attendance and exclusion of those with needs that do not match the target (Hughes, 1995).

A good example of structured, closed-end group work is the relatively short-term bereavement groups run by many hospices. In an article in *Bereavement Care* (1990) Broadbent et al. describe a structure that uses Worden's 'task'-based model of grief (1991) to support the content and process of group meetings. Explicitly sharing information about Worden's model also helps to reassure group members about the possibility of process and change and assists in removing some of the unhelpful 'elitism' surrounding professional knowledge.

Using Worden's 'tasks', initial meetings focus on *accepting the reality of the death* using 'story sharing' as a method of promoting trust. Members are then encouraged to *experience the pain of grief* through discussing experiences of dreams, depression, physical symptoms, guilt, regrets and so on. Powerful feelings are acknowledged and validated through the group process. Photographs are used to prompt memories. *The adjustment to an environment in which the deceased is missing* is tackled through talk about taking on new roles and decisions about managing issues such as scattering ashes and disposing of the deceased's personal possessions. A structured goodbye session aims to strengthen positive memories of the dead person, to discuss and encourage achievements, to emphasise that it is all right to do things differently and to begin to enjoy life again. Informal reunions can be encouraged by exchanging (with members' permission) names and addresses and a simple photostatted booklet of sayings, books, pieces of music and poems that have been found helpful by members could be distributed to all.

Referrals and selection process

How are members referred to the group – self-referrals, from colleagues, from other agencies? Adverts, posters? What information is required about possible members?

Various factors will determine the membership of the group, for example, number preferred for group, single sex, age range, culture, race.

There have been suggestions that the more group members have in common the more readily the therapeutic value of the group is accessed (Yalom, 1985). For instance, in the case of relationship to the bereaved person, groups for bereaved men, for bereaved adult children, for daughters, for older spouses, might all be categories of similarity. However the size of available client populations may determine membership, age, sex and ethnicity as well as particular problems to be focused upon. In any group being an 'only member', for example, the only male, black, or elderly person should be avoided where possible.

Facilitators need to consider what kind of behaviour they and other members of the group can cope with, for example, how safely can withdrawn or aggressive members be managed? They need to develop mechanisms to ascertain the individual's need for the group and their motivation to attend. In bereavement group work at St Christopher's Hospice potential group members are first written to and then screened by telephone call. Exclusion candidates might be those with a psychiatric illness, those already receiving some kind of one-to-one help, those who deny their own need for help or whose motivation appears to be that of instructing others in their own model of coping, for example, a fervent spiritualist. The screening process might also involve the length of time since the bereavement or particular kinds of bereavement. It is also important to give potential group members clearly written information about the purpose of the group, the time of meetings and their venue and any attendance commitments.

Leadership

Will there be one facilitator or two? If there is to be more than one facilitator, what kind of group culture and leadership style will they adopt? They will need time to talk to one another, to decide upon roles, to discuss issues of personal style around matters like self-disclosure. Time will also need to be set aside for *recording*, *debriefing* and *supervision* (who will provide the latter and how often?) These and other issues mean that group work is never primarily a resource-releasing activity. Facilitators will also need to discuss the content of sessions and how they will establish group rules. For example, at the one-off bereavement groups at St Christopher's Hospice group rules are defined as: confidentiality, maintaining time boundaries, one person only to speak at a time, respecting everybody's right to talk, and to start with, individuals introduce themselves by name and state their relationship to the deceased.

Practical resources

Practical issues that must be taken into consideration include the venue for the group (paying particular attention to issues of privacy), financial issues, transport, what sort of welcome will there be and how members who arrive early will be managed. Rooms will need to be large enough and equipment may be important. Refreshments are often significant in making people feel relaxed and cared for.

Liaison with colleagues and relatives

What information might be fed back and how? It is important to clarify the position for the group, explaining the rules surrounding confidentiality and any limits to them, while bearing in mind the follow-up for drop-outs from the group or the people it was decided should not attend.

Evaluation must also be considered

Will evaluation be conducted verbally at the end of the group or by later postal questionnaire or personal interview?

Ongoing group work for people with terminal illness

Interview with Frances Kraus, Principal Social Worker, St Christopher's Hospice, London

The setting is a well-established independent hospice with 62 in-patient beds and about 400 people being looked after at any one time in their own homes. The catchment area of St Christopher's Hospice is South-east London, ranging from inner city poverty to the affluent suburbs, with a considerable racial mix.

The group has been running for over five years and lasts for an hour. It has included people of various ages from 19 to 91 and from different races and sexual orientations. On average, 76 per cent of the participants are women and 24 per cent men, although at different times the group has consisted of all women and occasionally it has been mainly male. The group is for both in- and out-patients and has ranged in size from three to 15, with the average being seven members. The group meets in the family room at the hospice, which is set apart from both the main in-patient unit and the day centre, which is where the people who attend the group spend the rest of their day. This effectively increases the feeling of confidentiality and of being a group separate from other attendees at the day centre.

Breaking rules

Frances describes the importance of flexibility in group work with dying people. Many of the accepted principles of group work are not applicable to this group, for example, careful selection, commitment to regular attendance and punctuality. People fail to arrive because of unanticipated symptoms, exhaustion, clinic appointments or the vagaries of transport. All patients attending the day centre are made aware of its existence and choose whether or not to come for themselves. There is no automatic exclusion of people with difficulties in communication. On a number of occasions the group has included members with motor neurone disease who have used litewriters to communicate. The group has remained very tolerant of the inevitable time-lag in conversation.

Autonomy and flexibility

In the group, dying people themselves become both expert and therapist – their decisions and wishes are respected. The group is called 'the Thursday group' because the members involved at its inception did not want to be labelled 'the patients' group': 'We're people, not patients.' Since the group meets on a Thursday, this was the name they chose. The group was initially run for a series of eight fixed sessions. Members themselves requested the change to permanently ongoing weekly meetings. The group began as an open group, but its members decided they would like to return to the security of being a closed group. Very shortly members returned once again to an open group since the experience of people dying one by one and the group shrinking in size was distressing to all. The agenda is set by the group itself. As one of the group members commented, 'We talk about anything and everything and we don't talk about it outside.'

The role of the facilitator

Frances comments that one of the key roles of the facilitator is the maintenance of boundaries, for example, 'someone who starts and finishes the group on time regardless of members' arrival and departures' (Kraus, 1996). Frances also ensures that the group introduce themselves and explain how the group works and its rules whenever there is a new member. The group facilitator seems to provide a sense of safety and continuity in the presence of a constantly changing group membership. Group members also appreciate someone encouraging conversation and intervening when more than one conversation occurs at the same time. Frances makes explicit to group members one of the distinctions between conversations in the group and those that occur generally in the day centre: 'In the group we all listen to one person at a time and we don't talk about what has been said outside the group.' She comments that group members are reluctant to regulate this themselves and that they are content to let the facilitator maintain group discipline, often teasing her about behaving like a teacher. By taking control and managing the boundaries, the facilitator seems to encourage emotional release in the members.

Simple written information is given to potential group members: 'The Thursday group is for both in-patients and out-patients who would like the opportunity to talk about whatever matters to them in a relaxed setting.' Previous groups have been lively and caring and have included both humour and serious discussions. It is important to emphasise the role of the day centre in the success of the group. At the end of each meeting members retire to the day centre for a social lunch together, providing an automatic de-brief.

Overcoming anxieties

Prior to the formation of the group, staff expressed considerable anxieties about members becoming distressed and the worry that being with other people who were facing death would reinforce fears about their own mortality. The reality that terminally ill people were meeting one another informally anyway did not seem to affect this fear. Staff were also concerned that dying people would reveal important information about themselves and their families that would remain unavailable to staff members other than the group facilitators. Running the group initially for a series of eight sessions helped to alleviate anxieties as staff members could see that there would be a review point. Open discussion groups were also held where staff could express their anxieties, and research articles about the value of group work were circulated.

The group initially ran with two facilitators, but for several years there has been just one, the social worker attached on rotation to the day centre. The feeling at first was that two facilitators would provide more safety for the group, enabling it to continue if a member left upset and needed personal attention, and mutual support to the facilitators in what would be an emotionally demanding experience. Resource factors initially dictated the move to one facilitator, but the experience of running the group has been that it operates a subtle but extremely effective system of self-management, balancing painful topics with lighter ones. On the two occasions when members have left the group in distress another group member has immediately followed them. This was subsequently much appreciated not only by the distressed member but also by the helper who valued the opportunity to offer support.

Death of a group member

Another anxiety was that of talking to group members about the death of a fellow member. The facilitator tries to prepare the group when a member becomes less well, informing them of their progress. Frances describes waiting for a while after a session has begun before telling the group about a death so that members have started to come together as a group before hearing bad news. The group members usually spend time remembering the person who had died. We have asked group members about this experience and they frequently comment that it helps them to know that they, too, will be remembered (Monroe, 1997). One of the group members, a 40-year-old teacher, drew a clear distinction between friends and companions, commenting: 'As patients we are all up the same creek without a paddle. We live in a separate world. We are friendly towards each other, but we're not friends. We are companions. This is not painful, it is in fact warm and will support us as we undergo similar or joint experiences.'

Tolerance

Frances comments that tolerance is characteristic of the group, which often consists of members of different races, classes, education and life styles. The shared threat of serious illness in the group seems to transcend these differences and opposing views and opinions are expressed and accepted in a way that is rare in other social settings. Group members take risks with one another that would be very difficult for a member of staff. For example, one group member challenged another about confronting her teenager's difficult behaviour: 'Just go ahead and say it. You've got nothing to lose. Take your finger out.' There has been no evidence that anyone has been 'damaged' by this group. Members seem to be comfortable about deciding it is not for them. A few people do come once and not return, but on follow-up express no difficulty about this decision.

Group themes

Group themes include the illness itself, the shock of diagnosis, family relationships and the physical impact of such developments as incontinence and wearing wigs. Members have shared information about alternative therapies and their frustration about being dependent on others, for example, having to wait for someone to help them off the lavatory. They have argued about the power of positive thinking and depression, and the possibility and morality of suicide. Humour is often used as a coping mechanism – one member comforted someone else who was losing her hair by telling her about the time her own wig came off in the wind and she had to chase it down the road. The group will often balance a serious discussion by talking about a favourite topic such as holidays, food, television and the royal family.

Recording and evaluation

A record is kept of each group meeting, taking the form of a list of attendees and verbatim recording of significant comments and themes. The groups have usually been supervised within the individual supervision sessions offered to the social worker in the normal course of her work. The group has been evaluated from time to time by means of a simple questionnaire to group members. The question about how to best manage evaluation in the context of an ongoing group with constantly changing membership remains an open one. Comments have included: 'the value of being able to speak my mind', 'Realising that all the silly things I thought were unique to me happen to other people too, which made me calmer about myself', 'It made me realise I was quite well compared with other people.' Circulating the results of such evaluations to other staff members has helped to alleviate anxieties about the group.

Empowerment

One of the significant features of the group is that it reverses the dependence of the client upon the therapist, at least numerically. The group perhaps begs the question about whose fears we are really respecting, staff fears for patients or staff fears about their own mortality and authority. Facilitators comment that they have been more aware of the subtleties of people's personalities in the group than in any other situation. They become people, not patients, because they are relating to one another in an almost staff-free environment. The greater sense of power and autonomy conveyed by group membership has also been demonstrated in the frank criticisms of staff and the institution compared to the more usual anodyne replies to quality assurance questionnaires administered on a one-to-one basis. There has also been plenty of praise and appreciation. Frances describes running the group as an inspiring and exhilarating experience that has increased her knowledge and awareness and enriched rather than drained her emotional energy.

Single-session group work with bereaved children

Jenny Baulkwill, formerly Principal Social Worker, St Christopher's Hospice, London

Needs and objectives

Research indicates that unresolved childhood grief increases the risk of psychological problems in later life (Black and Young, 1995). Social workers at St Christopher's Hospice had had several years' experience of the value of adults sharing their experiences in single-session bereavement groups and wondered whether a similar approach might be helpful for children. (Such benefits have also been reported by Abeles, Oliviere and Pyke, 1995.) Joint case discussions had made them increasingly aware of the emotional isolation commonly experienced by bereaved children who, worked with individually, rarely seemed to have any significant contact with other children in similar circumstances apart from their own siblings (Smith and Pennells, 1995). Their parents were often so overwhelmed with their own grief that there was little opportunity for the sharing of emotional experiences within the family. A mutual protection often appeared to exist:

parents were anxious not to burden their children with their own feelings, whilst children expressed a fear of expressing feelings openly in case it hurt the parent. As one girl said: 'Maybe mummy wouldn't stop crying.' The group was intended to offer children the opportunity to meet and talk with other children in similar circumstances.

The general pattern of the group was to welcome the children, to help them feel part of the group and to get to know each other; to acknowledge their bereavement and explore what had happened in their families; to offer them a variety of opportunities to express their feelings; to share experiences together and to normalise their feelings, and help them to leave some of those feelings behind. The aim was also to give the children a good time (Baulkwill and Wood, 1994).

Selection and venue

The children invited are between 6 and 13 years old and attend the group session on a Saturday from 10.30 a.m. until 3.30 p.m. It was decided not to accept children without some experience of formal schooling in order to minimise the presence of those with difficulties in concentrating, in following instructions and in managing a long-day separation. Adolescents are catered for in a separate group. The wide age range has not caused difficulties, indeed the older children seem to enjoy helping younger ones. The venue is the hospice day centre which provides self-contained facilities with its own kitchen, toilet, sitting room and art room. Having the same physical environment for all the activities helps to avoid interruptions and contributes to maintaining the cohesion of the group. Adequate space is vital to allow for the release of energies and to work individually when required. Jenny commented that the first venue, a smaller, single room, proved cramped and led to more disruptive behaviour. Most of the children involved in the group come from families connected with the hospice, either through the in-patient unit or home care. Some of them will already have met a member of the social work department, others will not. Siblings have been accepted into the group as this was important to many of the parents – experience so far has not shown this to be a problem.

Setting the group up – ensuring safety

It has been important to have a high ratio of adults to children. The average group size has been eight children and the team has consisted of two social workers who act as group leaders, plus two experienced volunteer bereavement counsellors. The high staff/child ratio allows for the needs of each child to be addressed individually during some of the exercises and makes a vital contribution to the safety of the group. All parents or carers are sent a letter asking for permission to contact the children and explaining the purpose of the group. This is followed up with a phone call and a visit where necessary. The children then receive a separate illustrated invitation with reply slips and stamped addressed envelopes provided. It states specifically that they will be meeting and talking with others whose mother or father has died within the last year. It is important to give the children some sense of control over their response. The take-up rate for the group has been about 50 per cent.

The groups run on a Saturday during school term time, partly to allow free use of the day centre but also to avoid days in the holiday period when some children might be unable to attend. It has been possible to arrange transport to the group where necessary, because a one-off group has only represented a small burden on the volunteer transport force. The groups run on a rolling basis, one each school term. This means that professional staff know that they can refer children on a continuous basis, and that any delay will not be longer than two or three months.

Food has been an important part of the sense of security for children: 'grazing' food in the form of drinks, crisps, etc. is available throughout the day and food that is familiar but fun, such as ice cream with a variety of serve-yourself toppings and chocolate rice crispy cakes, have been popular for lunch.

Close working with parents has been very important. The death of a partner seems to revive separation anxieties. Parents are potentially handing their child over to an unknown adult, and the children, too, are anxious. It has been important to meet them at the door of the day centre so that they are physically helped over the threshold.

The shape of the day

Beginnings

Since the children inevitably all arrive at slightly different times it has been important to have a variety of small games and activities to keep them occupied while they wait until everyone has arrived. One of these activities is making and decorating their own name badges. There are drinks and biscuits available and music playing in the background. There is also a welcome board with all the children's names written on it. When the group proper begins the rules are stated, and written up: 'Most times are for talking and sharing. There are times to be quiet and listen. It's O.K. to cry, and it's O.K. to laugh and have fun' (Heegaard, 1988). One of the group leaders also makes a clear, simple statement acknowledging the reason for inviting the children and the purpose of the day, that all of them have had a mum or dad who has died. This links in with the invitation and its explicit message. There are then some ice-breaking games such as using a bean bag to throw to someone whilst saying their names.

Activities

The children next create a family tree with buttons. A large variety of different coloured, shaped and textured buttons is supplied and one of the group leaders demonstrates the process by developing her own family tree on a flip chart. The children are encouraged to draw whatever style of family tree they prefer, younger children often liking to literally draw a tree, older ones to make a structured chart. They are urged to include friends and pets and use blu-tack initially so that they can change the position of the buttons as they talk. The group leaders move between pairs of children helping them discuss their altered perception of where they are in their family and the changes that have happened to them. The children eventually stick the buttons down and can take their trees home at the end of the day. The children demonstrate a high level of imagination and concentration throughout this session. The information from it is not shared in the wider group and if siblings are present in the group they work separately from each other.

The next activity is around expressing and recognising feelings. The children brainstorm words for feelings. Then a piece of plain lining paper is cut to the height of each child and the child lays down on it and one of the helpers draws round them. The children think about their feelings in colours and where to put them in their bodies. Again the child can take their body art home. One mother wrote about moving house: 'During the move John took great care to keep the outline of his body and the memory jar safe.'

The children also show one another a photograph of the person who has died, which they were asked to bring in the invitation. A reassuring telephone call to the parent the day before the group also acts as a reminder about the photograph. The children are asked to say something special about their photograph and they then very freely ask one another questions: about what the person died of, how old they were, did they smoke, and so on. This activity is followed by the mystery suggestions box where each child is asked to write down something that has been helpful and something that has been unhelpful following the death of their parent. They post the papers in the box (a decorated shoe box with a slit in the lid) and each child in turn picks a paper from the box and either reads, or is helped to read, what is written and this is discussed in the group. Topics often focus around how the death was handled at school and peers' reactions to it, the funeral, anger about adults who say 'be brave' or 'I know how you feel' and the expression of emotion, whether or not it is good to cry. One boy wrote: 'My teacher made me tell the class what had happened, but I would of liked it if she told them' and a girl wrote: 'My computer teacher told everyone in my class that my dad had died without asking or telling me or my mum.'

Endings

At this point the two social workers leave the group of children to the two bereavement counsellors and run a separate group for the parents who have been asked to arrive an hour before the ending of the day, so that they can have a group of their own before taking their children home. During this time the children make a memory jar, colouring salt with chalks and filling an empty spice jar with layers of coloured 'memories'. This exercise encourages the children to recall positive memories of the dead parent. One child coloured the salt yellow: 'My mum made the best chips in the world.' It is followed by a candle ceremony using nightlights in memory of the person who has died, followed by a relaxation exercise.

The development of the parents' group has proved an important link between the children's group experience and their families. The group has usually run itself, with little prompting from the leaders. A great deal of pain is expressed about loneliness, physical exhaustion and role redefinition. Practicalities are discussed, for example, men talk about not knowing what bedtime stories to read and how to answer a child who keeps on saying: 'When are we going to see mummy again?' Many parents have spoken of the support given by this brief group experience and names and addresses are often exchanged.

When the parents and children reunite, the children are very excited and have the physical object of the memory jar to show their parent. Everyone then goes into the garden to release helium balloons. Jenny cautions workers to have several spares in case of burst balloons. As the balloons are released they think about a message and goodbye to the dead parent. It seems important that this activity is done with the parents. There is a reuniting and an expression of shared loss and shared goodbyes. At this stage things move swiftly towards the end. The children take with them their memory jars, family trees and body shapes. They are not letting go of everything, but the balloons have promoted a sense of release, of letting go some of the hurt and the togetherness makes the sadness bearable.

Obstacles

On a practical level there were only a few minor obstacles which were remedied fairly swiftly; these were finding the right venue and ensuring that catering and transport arrangements went smoothly. Jenny comments that perhaps the biggest obstacle in establishing the group was leaders' own anxieties. The majority of the social work department's contact with bereaved children had been on either an individual basis or indirectly through adult members of the family. As a result they lacked confidence in their group work skills with children and feared making things worse. However parents' written evaluations have affirmed the helpful nature of the experience for the children:

> Regarding the day itself, John really enjoyed it and it helped him a lot being with other children whose parent had died because, I think, he felt he wasn't different unlike with his friends at school. He talked a lot about what he had done and why and he talked quite openly (for John) about his feelings he had written down on the outline of his body, which he never said about before, even when asked. I must tell you that when John came home that day and talked so openly about his dad it was an enormous relief.
>
> Myself I knew there are other people who have suffered bereavement, but I was happy to hear that my feelings are felt by others. We were all experiencing the same things. I am no longer blaming myself, but comforting myself that it's normal following the death of a partner.

The key steps in realising the practice

Jenny emphasises the importance of:

- A careful initial approach to families in order not to de-skill parents at a very vulnerable time for them. They need full information and as much reassurance as possible
- Thorough preparation with particular attention to detail and timing
- Plenty of time for planning beforehand and feedback sessions both immediately after the group to share emotional pain, and then a short while later to discuss any children felt to be at particular risk and what kind of ongoing help should be offered to them
- The quickly established tradition of staff members taking off work the Monday after the group as a 'day in lieu', allowing time for reflection and relaxation
- A high ratio of staff to children to allow for individual attention
- Establishing the group rules at the outset makes clear the purpose of the day and the permission for different feelings to be expressed
- A variety of activities within a flexible structure, to allow the children to release emotions safely whilst maintaining discipline and sustaining their attention and interest
- The graduated programme with safe, built-in steps allows the children to feel comfortable in a group setting and the different mediums of self-expression help to provide variety, and develop the child's self-esteem and confidence.

Jenny comments on how important it is that developments to the group have been made in small stages, maintaining security so that the confidence of the families, the children and the workers has not been shaken. For example, the addition of the group for parents was a later development.

Possible further developments are a follow-up half-day, looking at the unresolved issues for that particular group, or perhaps a meeting with a doctor or nurse to ask any questions and using role plays to rehearse new approaches to difficult situations. Another idea under consideration is extending the parents' group to offer them the opportunity to do a memory jar, both for its therapeutic aspect and to provide another point of contact with their child's experience.

In conclusion Jenny comments that it is the children who give the group its significance, rather than what the facilitators are doing or saying. Hearing issues directly from other children has so much more meaning than a talk from an adult. As one little boy commented at the end of the day: 'The thing that makes you sad is when your mummy or daddy dies.' As with many other groups the common experience of the children seems to override any differences of class, culture or race.

A long-term closed group for young people

Pam Firth, Social Worker, Macmillan Runcie Day Hospice, St Albans

The Macmillan Runcie Day Hospice is a three-year-old purpose-built day hospice based in the grounds of the district general hospital. It is registered for use by 20 individuals per day for day care. The services available include a cancer information and support service, five Macmillan nurses operating an outreach service, the day hospice itself, psychosocial care from one social worker and a volunteer bereavement counselling service co-ordinated by a social worker/counsellor, which has an interesting contractual model with several groups of local GPs.

Philosophy

Our concept of self arises from the social experience of interacting with others. Pam asserts that since human beings spend most of their waking lives in groups and most human problems arise in groups, most difficulties can be worked out in groups, which give an opportunity for co-operative problem solving. Members of a therapeutic group are able to have an experience of being similar and different at the same time. This is particularly important for young people who are beginning to separate from their families and who need to identify strongly with their peers. Pam is concerned that people who have been social beings are often left to die alone and that those who are left may have to face their bereavement alone. Pam's group is designed to counteract this isolation and is clearly based on an experiential psychodynamic model, using an understanding of how individuals attempt to reconcile their inner thoughts and feelings with their outside reality.

The aims of the Young Persons' Group are to:

- Enhance social skills
- Improve self-esteem
- Reality test
- Help in managing strong feelings
- Develop interdependence to help with feelings of isolation
- Promote a sense of helping others as well as yourself
- Encourage talking out – not acting out.

Structure

The group runs on a Wednesday in term times from 4.15 to 5.45 p.m. The group size is usually about six and the groups have generally been for 13- to 16-year-olds, although 16- to 24-year-olds have also been catered for separately. The groups deliberately have a mix of bereavements, including both illness and sudden accidental death. Referrals are generated from the social worker's own contacts with families, from Macmillan nurses, bereavement counsellors and the contracting general practitioners. Once started, the group is closed. The group has two facilitators, Pam Firth herself and a colleague, often someone less experienced in group work from the local hospital social work team; recently the second facilitator was a Macmillan nurse. Pam emphasises that although one leader needs considerable group work experience, the second facilitator can be trained during the group itself on an apprenticeship model.

Beginnings

Most of the young people go home to change out of school uniforms before arriving at the hospice. There is an initial period of assembling which derives a ritual status from a cake made by a volunteer each week. This is known as 'Pauline's cake' and each week requests can be made for next week's preferred variety. Pop music is played in the background as group members arrive. This informal start helps the transition between school, home and the group.

Talking and playing

The group next moves on to a half-hour or more of talking time which is very much centred around the preoccupations that the young people bring with them, rather than a led discussion with themes emanating from the facilitators. They are prompted to talk about the good and bad things that have happened during the week. The facilitators' task is seen as picking up on key issues. The young people may decide to bring photographs of the dead person and talk about them, but this would be their decision. On one occasion, on their own initiative, they designed tombstones.

The session then moves into games playing (Brandes and Phillips, 1990). Pam comments on the young people's choice of regressive games. 'Twister', a game played on a mat where the body is contorted into difficult shapes, is a particular favourite that offers plenty of opportunity for release of energy. Another favourite game is building a balancing tower of bricks which then have to be pulled out one by one. This encourages talk about chaos, control, balance and family differences. Roulette also promotes talk about chance. One girl used it to reflect on her father's death in a helicopter crash. Board games about food are also popular and a video game with ghosts who direct the player to move tombstones on a games board is much liked. The ghost eventually turns into a skeleton and worms creep through it. Pam comments that this seems to respond to the young people's need for some process of confrontation with death. They use it as a prompt to talk about what it is like to visit the grave of a dead person and wonder about their rotting body.

Ending

The sessions end with the facilitators checking that the young people are content to leave and what they are going to do when they leave. The complete set of group sessions end with a symbolic ritual devised by the young people themselves. This has typically been an outing to a theme park. The young people do keep in touch with one another and often send messages to the facilitators about GCSE successes and so on.

Why run a group for young people?

Pam and the team noted that although they were aware of many bereaved young people in distress, most of them did not appear to accept offers of individual counselling. Groups are a natural environment for young people and she hypothesised that they might find an invitation to a group more attractive than the potential embarrassment and pressure of individual help. Just when young people need to feel part of their peer group, bereavement may make them feel very isolated and different. The group creates a temporary situation in which they can feel the same, a sort of short-term peer group which resolves the difficulty of isolation and permits exploration of difficult emotions. The young people are given a safe, formal place to talk about what is happening to them. Some talk readily in the discussions; others contribute little but their constant attendance indicate its helpfulness to them. They participate by listening and perhaps benefit from having some of their thoughts externalised by others. Young people like to help one another and peer affirmation is much more powerful than adult reinforcement.

Obstacles

Finding a good venue was a major obstacle to establishing the group. Prior to the building of the day hospice the group often had to meet in a number of different places during the life of one group. The young people's commitment to continued attendance despite these changes is a mark of the group's value to them. Once the new day hospice was established there were initial staff anxieties about unruly young people in a smart new building with new carpets and so on, as well as the manager's anxieties about insurance for potential damage. These were overcome by discussion but Pam comments that it is important to be realistic. The young people do have to be regularly reminded about limits to boisterous behaviour.

Key principles in establishing the group

A supportive management and team structure

Pam ensures a supportive structure by giving regular feedback to staff. She avoids group work being seen as a specialist social work function by using other members of the internal and external team as facilitators. Support from the external network has been vital to the group's success and using two facilitators who differ in terms of both their professional specialism and the agency for whom they work has also furthered general inter-agency co-operation.

An appropriate environment and suitable equipment

A room that is not too small, readily accessible and furnished in a warm and relaxing way is necessary. It needs a door that shuts to create a perceptible boundary and to afford considerable privacy. For example, Pam comments on the importance of blinds in the room she uses. The young people have decided that they like to sit round a table for their discussion, again emphasising the need for boundaries and security.

Equipment needs to be oriented toward quite a young age group: games, paper, puzzles, pens, etc.

Effective selection

Pam assesses potential group members individually, looking at need, motivation and capacity for engagement. She stresses that the young people really must want to attend and that it is important to ascertain that they are not being pushed by their families. Highly impulsive or acting-out youngsters are also excluded. Young people bereaved through suicide are not accepted for the group, as Pam thinks they might try to protect other members from such painful material.

Working with parents

A clear explanation to the young person and their family of how the group will work is vital to the success of the group. All parents are met personally prior to the group. They need to be reassured that the group workers are not going to form an alliance against them with the young people. They have to trust the facilitators' competence and the fact that they will not try to take over their parenting roles.

Confidentiality

The issue of confidentiality is vital if the young people are to feel safe to share their feelings. Parents and group members are told in advance that there is a rule of group confidentiality and that nothing will be passed on to parents without the young people's permission. Negotiated feedback has included discussion about trips and about writing to exam boards. However, Pam also makes it clear to the young people at the beginning of the group sessions that if the facilitators were seriously worried about a member, for example if he or she were talking about suicide or a dangerous piece of acting out, this would be reported back to parents. She says to them quite explicitly: 'I want to keep you safe while you are with us. I am responsible for you while you are in this building.' Recently the hospice has made a room available to any parents who want to stay during the 90-minute duration of the group. Tea, coffee and cake are provided but no specific staff members attend. The parents have welcomed this opportunity for informal conversation about their similar circumstances and difficulties.

Time for the facilitators

Pam emphasises the need for planning and personal discussion between the facilitators, immediate sessional de-briefs and planned external supervision. Thematic notes are taken of each group and used in supervision. She comments wryly that the group work is not a cheap alternative. She estimates that the two facilitators each spend three to four hours per week in total on the group.

A mission statement

Each new series of groups begins with the group itself generating its rules and a mission statement through a brainstorm. The following extra rules also apply: no physical violence, no damaging property, tidying up afterwards and time limits.

Long-term group work

The length of the groups (most of them run for three school terms) has been a source of surprise to Pam and her colleagues. They initially thought that young people would only agree to something relatively short term, not too committed. Initially the members are told that the group will run for a term and that its continuance will be negotiated at the end of each term. They are told that it will not last for longer than a year. All group members have requested that the group continue after the first term.

Pam observes the following phases in the group:

1. *Early phase*

   - Group dependent on leader building up attachment.
   - Pairing often happens.
   - Identification of group norms.

2. *Middle phase*

   - Role differentiation is seen.
   - More sharing of strong feelings and an interchange of experience.
   - It becomes possible for the members to accept feedback.

3. *Later phase*

   - Degree of closeness has been established.
   - Revisiting losses in safety.
   - Issues about leaving the group and needing support to separate.

What is distinctive about group work with young people?

Pam underlines the need to move quickly once an appropriate number of bereaved young people have been identified. Over-preparation can diminish the facilitators' confidence so that they almost talk themselves out of running the group. Young people themselves will not wait around; moods, enthusiasms and themes change quickly and have to be caught and worked with while they are fresh. A strong container needs to be provided if young people are to feel safe enough to express powerful and sometimes primitive feelings. There needs to be considerable thought about boundary activity: beginnings, endings, the mucking about that takes place at the end of each group and the need to hand the young people over to their families who are going to transport them home. There is more interplay with the family and great attention has to be paid to this.

Future plans

For the future Pam wonders about meeting the needs of bereaved parents with a very long-term parent circle meeting once a month. She comments on the difficulty of parenting a bereaved child whose bereavement continues and changes throughout their growing up. She thinks that as the struggles are long term, perhaps group work also needs to be long term. Parents might value informal peer support, for example, being able to talk about the experience of having to choose a secondary school for your child on your own. She would also like to improve links with other agencies and is collaborating with a new young people's counselling service by being a voluntary director of the service.

Group work in palliative care

The three groups described illustrate different methods of group work. They also demonstrate different leadership styles which could be crudely characterised as *laissez-faire*, authoritarian and democratic. Methods need to be appropriate to the aims of the group, but leadership style is also highly dependent for its success on its congruence with the personality, values and existing practice of the worker. An adequate level of comfort and confidence in the leader is vital in order to convey to group members the necessary sense of safety that paradoxically permits risks to be taken.

All of the groups demonstrate the importance of clear aims and careful preparation. Their 'success' is most readily defined by the participants' enthusiastic commitment to attendance at group sessions. However the actual duration of the session is merely the visible culmination of a much greater proportion of planning and consultation time.

Hard data on long-term outcomes is not available either for the three groups used in this chapter or for most other pieces of group work. However, their simple evaluations reveal expected gains in lessening of isolation, emotional release through discussing painful feelings with others in a similar situation and an increased understanding of the variety of responses to loss and some practical ways of managing its inevitably stressful impact. In a fascinating article on 'The challenge of evaluating a child bereavement programme', Stokes, Wyer and Crossley (1977), reflect on the difficulties of identifying appropriate measures and of deciding what it is that we really want to measure. As Silverman and Worden emphasise (1993): 'Bereavement outcomes need to be conceptualised in more dynamic terms that emphasise change and adaptation rather than merely the presence and absence of symptoms or signs of psychological disturbance.' Stokes describes an interesting experiment using a letter format with incomplete sentences to elicit the family's own perception of the Winston's Wish Camp and its effects: 'When ... died it was hard because ...', 'At camp I liked ...', 'I did not like ...', 'Since camp, these things have changed ...'.

All facilitators of groups in palliative care settings stress the particular importance of strong boundary management given the explosive and painful mixture of feelings and anxieties surrounding loss and death. Beginnings and endings become particularly important. Each session's end can be experienced as a separation and may echo how people are coping with their major loss. The end of any session must allow time for group members to feel safe enough about the content of the session and to become ready to move away and on to the next activity of their day. The end of a series of sessions may offer an opportunity to model a more contained and planned ending than that of the actual loss.

Perhaps the key messages for group work are:

- Feel enthusiastic and ready to have a go
- Think ahead
- Get the beginning right
- Recognise the need for supervision
- Have a working model and be prepared to change it in the light of experience
- Recognise the importance of endings.

5 Gender and sexuality

'With a few exceptions, there are two sexes, male and female ... Gender is a term that has psychological and cultural rather than biological connotations.'
(Stoller, 1968)

'Age, ethnicity, gender, social class and sexuality all profoundly affect the ways people experience death, dying and bereavement.'
(Field, Hockey and Small, 1997)

Gender and sexuality largely determine the person. Why are gender and sexuality important in palliative care? A specialty, devoted to operating a very personalised service in respecting the unique nature of the ill person and family, must know how to work with gender issues and sexuality: how men and women cope with loss; self-image and self-esteem as the body deteriorates; dying and grieving and their impact on intimacy, and the specific needs of gay and lesbian people are just some of the areas that need consideration for good practice in psychosocial palliative care.

One cannot work holistically without integrating gender and sexuality into one's thinking, although, as in many aspects of our work, the issues are sensitive and delicate and are often addressed as part of other issues. As with culture, the perception of gender and sexuality is filtered through the gender and sexuality of the professional, the lens through which patient and carer is focused. In addition to multi-professional teamwork in palliative care, it is also recognised that in practice if a broad discussion involving different gender perspectives is held, a more balanced decision may result (Randall and Downie, 1996).

At a practice level, one needs to be aware of the effect of our behaviour and that of society and its differing impact on men and women – from 'observations that ... adult men of working age receive greater attention from hospital staff and are far more likely to be told their terminal diagnosis than women, especially old women' (Field, Hockey and Small, 1997), to the fact that men do not receive the equivalent to Widowed Mother's Allowance.

It has been shown that women experience disadvantage at the end of life both as dependants and carers. More of the people who are most dependent live alone, with few sources of informal care and these tend to be women. Women are most likely to take on the main burden of caring, particularly where they are spouses, who are often themselves elderly with health problems. These same women are amongst those most likely to be living alone after the death, the greater number of women surviving their husbands (Seale and Cartwright, 1994).

'Gender' and 'sexuality' are two separate but overlapping entities. No strict distinction is made for the purposes of examining palliative care practice: 'Sexuality is an integral part of every human being ... it is more than a physical expression, it is about self-concept, self-esteem and social role, which combine to form the identity of the person' (Poorman, 1983). 'Intimacy, the ability to communicate and receive love, of which sexual intercourse itself is only one part, is a vital human need ... Cancer changes the way people feel about themselves and each other' (Monroe, 1993a).

With HIV/AIDS, as it is frequently a sexually transmitted condition, 'infection with the virus can lead to an unwelcome examination of sexual behaviour and curtailment of previously enjoyed behaviour, and may mark periods of abstinence, psychosexual hurdles and problems. This comes at the very time when the expression of close, loving intimacy may be especially desired' (Sherr, 1995).

The practices described in this chapter demonstrate a gendered and sexual approach to palliative care. The importance of the practices lies in the greater consciousness of gender and sexuality within psychosocial palliative care and in treating people as fully human. Although much discussed in society, gender and sexuality are only addressed in the palliative care literature in a very limited way. It is impossible to discuss gender issues without acknowledging their wider context in society: the social construction of gender identity and inequalities between the sexes embodied in language and institutions.

A sexual-sensitive approach to palliative care

Interview with Barbara Monroe, Director of Social Work, St Christopher's Hospice, London

St Christopher's Hospice (see Chapter 3), has pioneered teaching about sexuality as part of its multi-professional training programme.

What do you mean by sexuality?

In an article for the *Journal of the Royal College of General Practitioners*, Judy Gilley commented, 'A search of the literature on terminal illness shows it to be singularly lacking in references to sexuality and its implications for terminal care' (Gilley, 1988). Ten years on, the situation is not much improved. Gilley defines sexuality as 'the capacity of the individual to link emotional needs with physical intimacy'. Most of us would accept the need of all human beings to communicate and receive love and that this is done in a variety of ways. Sexual intercourse is only one part of a whole language of intimacy and should not be over-emphasised. As they approach death, people's need for physical closeness, to touch and be touched, to stroke, to hug, may be much more significant in terms of quality of life. Palliative care has always stressed the holistic approach, the determination to meet physical, spiritual, social and emotional needs. Professionals working in the area must, therefore, have some commitment to helping patients and their partners and those close to them with their sexual needs.

In a study of young women with cancer of the cervix, Vincent et al. (1975) reported that 80 per cent of those receiving treatment wanted more information about the impact of the disease on their sexuality. However 75 per cent of them said they would not raise the question first. Sexuality remains a 'no go' area both for those in receipt of care and for the professionals delivering that care. The combination of sexuality and palliative care is a powerful one, presenting us with two taboo subjects. Most professionals share most individuals' common difficulty in talking about their own sexuality. The combination of sex and death has a potent power to break down the barriers between professional and private individual that we erect to keep us safe. The subject reminds us of our non-professional selves, of our own needs and uncertainties. Sexuality is not 'their' problem, safely at one remove, it is ours too. All teams have a responsibility to educate and train themselves in the area of sexuality. In order to do this they will need:

- To increase their awareness of their own sexuality so that they can hear the issues of their clients rather than the assertions of their own norms
- To increase their awareness of others' sexuality
- To explore professional boundaries and limits
- To develop knowledge of the physical effects of illness upon sexuality
- To develop knowledge of the emotional and psychological effects of serious illness and bereavement upon sexuality
- To become more able to discuss sexuality with others, to help them to articulate and share their problems and needs
- To become more aware of the institutional dyamics involved and to generate ideas for improving service delivery.

It must be emphasised that we are not talking about training specialist counsellors in psychosexual needs, but about practitioners who are comfortable with offering and responding to cues about sexuality. If sexuality is to become an integral part of the clinical routine, health and social care professionals must be trained to identify and to assess need, to initiate dialogue and discussion and to offer first-line help.

Do practitioners need to explore their own sexuality before discussing that of others?

This is a major issue for any training. It is important for course members to begin to explore where they acquired their knowledge of sexuality. Our own understandings are likely to be biased by where and how we learnt about sexuality. In a survey reported in the *Guardian* on 28 March 1994, the Schools' Health Education Unit questioned 29,000 children aged 11 to 16. Although more than half of them thought that their parents ought to be their main source of information, most obtained it from their friends. This led to inevitable mythologising and gaps in information and knowledge. There was, for example, widespread ignorance about what birth control services were available locally (*Guardian*, 1994). Each of us would place different sexual activities on a continuum from acceptable to unacceptable in a different way according to our beliefs. We need to understand that the range of beliefs is wide and often strongly held. The important point for practice is not that professionals must condone or wish to share an individual's particular view of sexuality, but that they should wish to understand its significance for that individual.

A training exercise that helps practitioners to think about such issues is putting together small groups preferably of mixed professionals and issuing them with a range of cards containing the name of a particular sexual practice, for example: pre-marital sex, oral sex, anal sex, pornography, indecent exposure, prostitution, and asking them to place them on the floor in order of acceptability. Each student places their own card between plus and minus markers. They then go round their group each stating which placed card they find most unacceptable and where they would like to move it to and why. When a group of bereavement volunteers did this exercise one of them was finally able to confront her own absolute disgust for oral sex and to begin to talk about the fact that her now divorced husband had insisted on her joining in this practice, which she had found degrading. Her anxiety about a client raising this issue had made her fearful to discuss sexuality in any way with any of the people she was trying to help.

Another training idea that has proved useful is to show participants on the course a video of profoundly physically disabled people talking about their sexuality. This is followed by a discussion in pairs of the challenges presented by the video to the individual when thinking about their own sexuality. Issues raised include the difficulty of imagining sexuality in any way as appropriate to such profoundly disabled people, or revulsion at the thought of personally engaging in a sexual act with one of the individuals. Opening up the discussion in this way has helped professionals to move forward to a greater awareness of the importance for everyone of the acceptance of their sexual being. It can also sometimes help simply to ask participants to turn to the person next to them and to discuss whether or not they shave their armpits and whether or not they prefer shaved or unshaven armpits. Many of our sexual expectations are societally engineered. A discussion of acceptable sexual images and their power is also useful. How does it feel to be an individual with cancer, perhaps to have had treatment that has caused hair loss, constantly assaulted by television and magazine commercials for shampoos that portray the image of a sexually acceptable person as someone with long, glossy, beautiful hair?

All such discussions must include thinking about gay male relationships and lesbian relationships. For some groups it will be important to give simple information about what may be physically involved in such relationships as they may lack such knowledge and fear of exposing their own ignorance may cause them to avoid the subject altogether.

The professional's own assumptions can deny individuals the help they need. A young couple may be offered a double bed and an individual room in a hospice. Are the same facilities always considered for an elderly couple to whom they may be equally important? The assumption may be made that the young unmarried woman does not have a partner – perhaps her female visitor feels too frightened of being judged to reveal that they are indeed sexual partners, rather than just flatmates. The loss of what we have never had is also a potent issue. Professionals who themselves have not experienced sexual intercourse may feel reluctant to discuss it with others. Equally we should remember the power of the statement by a 14-year-old boy with an incurable sarcoma: 'I've never even screwed a girl.'

Are there not professional boundaries and limits as to what can be undertaken?

Rights and respect need to be operated on both sides of the professional/client boundary. Staff who are involved in the intimate care of ill people and those close to them need to think in advance about the issues. Nurses who gave much appreciated cucumber massages to a middle-aged man with motor neurone disease should not perhaps have been so surprised when his wife became aggressive and jealous of his pleasure in their attention. It might have been better for them to train her in delivering the massage. Equally, professionals infringed the right to personal respect of a young man with a brain tumour when they over-responded to him physically in a way that was consistent with the intellectual level that he *appeared* to demonstrate in his much reduced verbalisation and disinhibited behaviour. Staff cuddled and petted him, but became disturbed and annoyed when he began to touch them inappropriately, trying to unbutton their blouses and touch their breasts. He was a sexually active young man in his mid-twenties and needed respect for the whole of who he was.

Professional staff also need to feel comfortable with declaring their own rights when their boundaries are infringed. A young woman doctor in training in palliative care was completely dumbfounded during a home visit to a man with terminal cancer when he looked at her and said: 'Please hold my penis.' Unable to think how to respond she did so and then felt very awkward about letting go of the penis. The discussion that ensued in the staff team later was helpful to all. We all need to know that it is acceptable to say 'No, I can't do that, but I do want to understand why you asked me that. It sounds as if this is something that is very important to you.' The bereavement volunteer who is asked questions such as 'Are you married?' or 'Would you come out and have a drink with me sometime?' needs to have the opportunity in training and supervision to discuss appropriate responses, for example, 'I am here as your counsellor, not your friend, but I do want to talk about things that are important to you, the things that hurt you and leave you feeling alone and empty.' Left undiscussed in training, such issues can become major inhibitors in practice. In an exercise around brainstorming 'nightmares' during a training course on sexuality, people spoke about how to manage being attracted to a client themselves and the difficulties of responding to people who 'try it on' by making statements such as 'Do you know that you are very attractive?' Also, anxieties are discussed concerning colleagues or relatives misinterpreting therapeutic touch. For example, an aromatherapist revealed that several colleagues had repeatedly asked the question 'Aren't you getting a bit too involved?' Further 'nightmares' including being afraid of embarrassment when the bereaved widow finally, and with much difficulty, asks you 'Is it all right to masturbate?'

Knowing how to continue the conversation or just being frightened of being asked a question to which you do not know the answer, needs rehearsal. As in many other areas of practice, professionals need reminding that we do not have to know all the answers, that for many people just to discuss the issues would be sufficient and that we can always offer to find out more or to refer them on to someone with more expertise if this is appropriate and acceptable to the individual.

What specific areas of knowledge do practitioners require?

Knowledge of the physical effects of serious illness

Both surgery and treatment can result in what might be crudely called 'mechanical' sexual problems. For example, radical vulvectomy removes the clitoris, radical hysterectomy shortens the vagina. Removal of the prostate may cause a man to have dry ejaculations in which semen goes into the bladder and the sensation may be that ejaculations are different. The removal of tumours of the rectum can cause problems with erection (Gill, 1997).

Equally important, however, are the changes that serious illness can cause in the way people feel about themselves and their sexuality (Jaffe, 1979; Fallowfield, 1992). Crowther, Corney and Shepherd (1994) comment that what makes sexual dysfunction 'so difficult to treat is its psychogenic component'. As they remind us in their article about gynaecological cancer, 'surgery to the breast and genitals threatens female identity. The disruption of body image, particularly from the mutilating surgery of radical vulvectomy ... results in many women never resuming intercourse.' The emotional and physical consequences of illness are closely linked together. Professionals need to understand the direct physical consequences of illness and treatment to be able to help partners with issues about 'how do we do it when it is difficult or painful?'

They also need to understand the changes wrought by illness in the way people feel about themselves and each other. This will include difficult issues such as physical repulsion and guilt. In the extremely helpful book *Sexuality and Cancer* (1995) written by Dr Andrew Stanway for BACUP, he categorises how cancer and its treatments affect sexual responses: 'Disorders of desire, pain, surgery, radiation therapy, chemotherapy and hormone therapy'. Depression and anxiety can decrease desire and the fatigue, nausea, diarrhoea, skin rash and so on that accompany treatment can also make sex and feeling alive sexually more difficult. Many such mechanical difficulties can be reduced or eliminated with effective sexual counselling (Capone et al., 1980).

Information about anatomical changes and alternative sexual techniques needs to be clearly and simply communicated to patients, and partners if appropriate. The use of drawing and diagrams can help. Other ways of expressing themselves sexually can be suggested, for example, mutual masturbation or alternative positions. Such discussions need to be offered pro-actively by the health care professional and ideally in advance of any such treatment. For example, women receiving pelvic radiation can be advised to use vaginal dilators with lubricating jelly, or to have regular intercourse or to use their own or a partner's fingers to gently flex the vaginal area. The impact of steroid therapy on physical appearance needs discussing wherever possible, not only with the individual but with the partner. Professionals can also give ill individuals copies of the BACUP and Cancerlink booklets that are available (Cancerlink, 1993, 1995a).

Knowledge of the institution

The physical barriers erected by institutions also need consideration. These take a variety of forms, from the availability of single rooms and double beds, to the sensitivity with which staff are trained to raise such issues and the general levels of acceptance and permissiveness that the institution as a whole seems to generate.

At one hospice a 42-year-old woman who had enjoyed a vibrant sexual life with her dying partner was adamant that she wanted to get him home in order that they could resume the physical intimacy that had been so important a part of their relationship. When offered a single room at the hospice she replied with incredulity, 'You mean fuck him here? Impossible. It's like a church.' General privacy is vital as is respect and attention to the detail of people's physical care.

Detailed attentiveness and care for appearance may be vital for the ill person. One elderly lady with terminal cancer was given a very unattractive haircut by a well-meaning volunteer; she reported that that was the thing that made her feel as if she just wanted to give up. Hospices now increasingly employ professionally trained hairdressers and aromatherapists, recognising the enormous enhancement of people's sense of physical well-being that such services can provide. All units should endeavour to provide both relevant booklets and information sheets with details of both local and national resources, e.g. the Association to Aid the Sexual and Personal Relationships of People with a Disability, Relate for relationship counselling, local psychosexual counsellors and clinics and shops selling suitable aids and material and their postal services.

Knowledge of the emotional and psychological consequences of serious illness and bereavement on sexuality – 'How can we be close again?'

The physical difficulties caused by surgery and treatment for serious illness can be considerably exacerbated by myths, fears and false expectations. Questions such as : 'Is cancer contagious?' or 'Is cancer a punishment for some previous sexual activity?' can feel difficult to ask and difficult to answer. A partner may be anxious about sex causing pain or harm or worry that sex will sap much-needed strength. Injunctions to generations of sportsmen have done nothing to diminish this particular myth.

Then there are feelings on both sides about changed body image, for example, hating the way one's body looks now, or a partner feeling anxious about whether they can accept the changed image of an ill partner. A vicious circle of false expectations and misunderstanding can quickly set in. Both partners may be ill at ease, lacking in self-confidence, angry and depressed. Anxiety about rejection can put a strain on existing relationships and make it very hard to make new ones. An example could be a woman who has just had a mastectomy; her partner's assurances that 'sex doesn't matter, you're alive, that's all that's important' can be misinterpreted as repulsion. In order to avoid the pain of this, the ill person may rebuff any advance by her partner assuming it to be motivated by pity. This can lead to the partner's retreat and a wall of silence may develop that can be made worse by professional avoidance. Individuals and those close to them need time to talk and to come to terms with their illness and its implications. A colostomy may cause anxiety about smell and leakage, a hysterectomy raises issues about loss of fertility. All can be at least eased by discussion. Everyone needs reassurance that good sex is built on good communication, not good bodies. As Dr Stanway comments in *Sexuality and Cancer*: 'However bad the effects of treatment, people with loving partners who can communicate with each other and explore sexually pleasurable activities can still enjoy fulfilling sex, even if what goes on in the bedroom is rather different than before.'

It can assist enormously if a health care professional suggests to a couple that when trying to get back to sex it often helps to avoid penetrative sex as a focus or a goal, at least initially, focusing rather on physical caresses and erotic activities. Of course it is also true that people bring with them to serious illnesses all the issues that were present for them as a couple before.

Practice example

Sally and Paul had been married for 26 years and had two adult children. Sally was 46 and was referred to the Home Care Team with a cervical cancer for which no more treatment could be given. She had been admitted to the in-patient unit for two weeks to examine her symptom control. On the ward she burst into tears and told the social worker 'I'd just love to be closer to Paul.' Sally revealed that she was brought up by elderly parents and had always been frightened of sex. She had never enjoyed intercourse with her husband who only seemed aware of his own needs. After the children were born she tried to put him off as much as possible. Since the cancer was diagnosed Paul no longer even kissed Sally. She felt very lonely. When she tried to touch Paul he just shrugged her off. Sally agreed to an offer that the social worker talk to Paul on his own. He said 'Sally never wanted sex, now she's just teasing me. We've never shared any interests. I'm happy to look after her but I'm finished with all that love business. I'd rather go for a game of golf.' Sally and Paul both resisted joint interviews. They did, however, agree to some sharing by the social worker with each of them as an individual acknowledging the other's faults and difficulties. Sally eventually died in the in-patient unit, with Paul visiting her regularly and helping in some aspects of her physical care such as brushing her still beautiful hair. They never, however, came to any intimate physical understanding or demonstrable affection.

What are the main factors relating to sexuality in bereavement?

While sex is often a problem after bereavement there have been few attempts to study the subject. A welcome exception to this is an article, 'Sexual needs of those whose partner has died' by Brenda Elliott in *Bereavement Care*. Elliot describes the confused nature of many widows' sexual behaviour: 'When erotic feelings do return they may come unexpectedly ... often accompanied by guilt' (Elliott, 1979). It may seem to the bereaved individual as if sex is the only way to achieve closeness. They may find themselves having unaccustomed quick affairs that leave them feeling confused and guilty. Equally, some of their desire for closeness, their acute physical yearning, can lead others to misinterpret their cues and assume that their desires are for sexual intimacy rather than physical closeness. The bereaved of both sexes may have to relearn sexual behaviours that have become unaccustomed, such as flirting. Those with little sexual experience before marriage may fear impotence and loss of control on the loss of a sexual partner, along with confusion and self-doubt about whether they can be sexually attractive to someone else. When the bereaved do find new partners they may be beset by the anxieties of others, particularly adult children, who are shocked at the sexual activity of their bereaved parent and concerned about its seeming lack of loyalty to a dead parent. Older people may be anxious about masturbation (Malatesta et al. 1988).

A bereavement can also create different sexual responses in an otherwise strong partnership. For example, parents who experience the loss of a child may find that they both have very different attitudes (Schwab 1996). The mother may not wish to have sex as it seems wrong to engage in an act of potential procreation whilst actively grieving the loss of a child. For her husband, the father of that dead child, sex may be his only way of achieving comfort, closeness and a sense of being alive in the middle of misery (Hagemeister and Rosenblatt, 1997). Counsellors need to be aware of the modifying process of bereavement on sexual needs and learn the skills to raise and discuss these issues with clients. Two quotes from Susan Wallbank's helpful book *The Empty Bed* summarise the issues: 'The passionate early days of being in love are very similar to the passionate painful days of grief' and 'Nothing offers a greater sense of safety and security than the know-ledge that we are joined to another living human being' (Wallbank, 1992).

What part does culture play in sexuality?

Culture also affects all aspects of sexuality and anxieties about ignorance of cultural and religious practices can further inhibit professionals' exploration of the area with very ill people. It is perhaps particularly important to offer individuals same-sex counsellors, but then gentle questioning with a clear request for permission remains the sensible way forward, for example, 'I'm not sure how important an issue this is for you at the present time or how comfortable you would feel to discuss it with me, but I'd like to ask you whether your illness has raised any sexual questions or issues for you or your partner.' As with any conversation about sexuality it is particularly important in such discussions to reassure the individual about the confi-dentiality of the conversation. Sometimes in palliative care it is the professionals' responsibility to protect a vulnerable ill person from the unwanted sexual attentions of partner.

How can practitioners help?

Remember sexuality is part of the person

Perhaps the most important reassurance for professionals working in this area is to emphasise that they will be using their existing skills in working with issues of sexuality. Because it is hard for us to talk about our own bodies, our own sexuality and sexually active selves, we often isolate the whole area of sexuality to one that requires a particular 'specialism'. The reality is that the communication skills required are the same for approaching any other sensitive topic. The professional needs to give infor-mation (often in advance of it being requested), to anticipate fears, to explore expectations, to normalise and reassure.

Listen for cues

One of the most important skills is being able to recognise the cues that vulnerable individuals give us when they are trying to test out whether we are safe enough and prepared enough to discuss such a personal topic with them. Examples of such cues are: the woman aged 55 dying from cancer of the cervix who said of her partner 'He just doesn't seem to love me any more'; the 65-year-old man with cancer of the lung who said to a nurse caring for him 'My erections embarrass me'; the wife of a man aged 58 with cancer of the bladder, 'He won't even let me kiss him'; and the 20-year-old boyfriend of a 19-year-old woman with cancer of the cervix: 'I just don't fancy her any more'; or the still-attractive 45-year-old woman with cancer of the breast: 'Before the cancer I felt young and sensual – now I am a fat, bald, one-breasted old woman.' All too often, faced with such shyly uttered statements the professional retreats into bland reassurances like 'Oh, I am sure he does love you', or changes the subject swiftly. Such responses serve to confirm individuals in their worst fears and suspicions that this subject is indeed too dangerous and too painful to discuss.

Invite openness through the general and specific

All staff need training in screening for sexual problems and issues as they would screen for uncontrolled symptoms, spiritual needs, family support needs or financial needs. It often helps to use questions that move from the general to the specific and that imply in their phrasing the acknowledgement that many people experience these kinds of doubts and insecurities: 'How has your illness/treatment affected your work/home/sex life? Do you have any worries about the sexual side of things?' Or certain statements can help, for example, 'People often have questions they would like to ask about the sexual side of life.'

Examples of sensitive questioning

A typical history might include the following sorts of questions:

- How long have you been together?
- Has the physical side of your relationship been important to you/your partner?
- How were things for you before the illness?
- How have things changed?
- In what ways has your illness changed the sexual side of your relationship?
- In what ways has your illness changed the way you can get close to your partner, to your friends, to your family?
- Have you coped with times like this before?
- What do you want most from your partner at the moment?
- What would help you most? Is there any way I could help you with that?
- What do you think your partner's reaction would be?
- How do you think you could get closer?

It is important to seek clarification: 'Can you tell me a bit more about that?' 'When did that first happen?' 'What happened after that?' 'How did that make you feel?' 'Did anything make it better/worse?' 'Has anything like this ever happened before in your relationship?' 'How did you deal with it then?'

It is important to notice disparities in verbal and non-verbal messages and vital to find a shared vocabulary. Some individuals are more comfortable with anatomically correct language, others prefer to use slang. The professional must enquire sensitively and be alert to clues. It is important to offer people the chance to talk alone and together if that is what they want. Working with partners in these areas raises for all health care professionals the acute but often ignored differences between talking to an individual and talking to partners or family.

Practice example

June was 40 and her partner, Patrick, 42; they were both teachers. They had been together for ten years and had two young sons aged six and four. June had advanced and incurable cancer of the breast, diagnosed just after her youngest son's birth. She had had two mastectomies on different occasions and now had bony metastases. She was thin, intermittently in a lot of pain, nauseated with poor balance and very little hair following her last lot of chemotherapy. She was under the home care team. A visit to her and Patrick together, had lasted almost an hour focusing mostly on the needs of the children and ways of involving them appropriately in what was going on in the family. June had also discussed how fed up and resentful she had been feeling towards Patrick nagging her to eat more: 'I know he cares, but it is so unhelpful.' Patrick was tense and distracted and had been trying to persuade June to get a nanny to help with child care. She was extremely resistant to this. While the social worker was talking to them both June suddenly unexpectedly asked: 'Have you got any ideas for improving our sex life?'

Sometimes it is appropriate to share the obvious response: 'You've taken me by surprise, I can see this is an important issue for you.' Because in this case the professional is talking to a couple it is important to then check out whether the other partner also wants to discuss this. It could be, for example, that he did not want to have a sex life, let alone improve it: 'Are things the same for you, Patrick?' In the actual instance the reply was yes, so the worker then asked: 'When do you get the time and space to make love at the moment? What is actually more difficult now?' Suggestions about alternative positions, the use of pillows, music and some wine were all received gratefully, but even more importantly the opportunity to talk about what a central part of their lives together, the act of making love, had been and continued to be.

The salutary reminder for the professional was that she had not even considered that this couple were continuing to have a sexual life. Humour will alleviate the embarrassment in many situations: 'I bet you'd never thought you'd find yourself talking to a relative stranger about a subject like this' or, 'I often go red when I'm talking about sex, just ignore me.'

Realism is vital. We cannot cure or heal all the wounds from the past.

Practice example

Peter was 49 with multiple myeloma. His wife, Kay, looked thin and exhausted. They had two teenage children. Peter said that he was sleeping in the spare room: 'The spenco fits the bed better, doesn't it Kay?' Kay looked away The atmosphere was very tense as Peter said to the counsellor: 'I tell her every night I love her and she says nothing.' The counsellor's job is not to indulge in unnecessary confrontation but to move the couple to the point where they realise that they have a choice both as a couple and as individuals and that the responsibility for acting on that choice is theirs. As in other work with couples, it is important to try to find common ground, but also to be aware of unspoken issues. The worker in this case looked to Peter and said quietly: 'You sound very lonely' and then looked over to Kay's back and said 'You look very lonely, too, Kay. Things feel very tense. Is there something you'd like to talk about?' The silences continued between each statement of the worker. The worker eventually said: 'Illness brings a lot of changes, sometimes it makes already painful things more difficult. It can help to talk. You might like to talk to me individually, or together.' The silence persisted. Peter was then asked if he would like to talk. He said yes, on his own, and Kay said similarly. Talking to them individually revealed the following. Peter felt lonely and frightened. He had always taken the decisions in the relationship and now longed for physical affection and reassurance. He wanted to be back in the double bed. Kay never seemed to want to touch him. He didn't want to impose. She had so much to do already and he worried that he was repulsive. He said that he felt 'half a man'. Kay described herself as exhausted. Peter was going to die, she would have to struggle on with the children. Everything was uncertain, including Peter's prognosis. She was just trying to get on with his care. She didn't want to think about him as a person, it was less painful to regard him as the patient. She said 'Sex is the last thing on my mind.'

With help this couple were eventually able to begin to share their anxieties with one another. Kay became more physically affectionate with Peter, although they never again shared a double bed.

Key issues in working with sexuality

- Individuals will not ask for help spontaneously. Learning to ask is the professional's responsibility.
- Don't make assumptions.
- Anticipation and honest discussion can reduce anxiety.
- Give reassurance.
- Offer privacy, time and warmth.
- Remember people's needs to be seen separately and alone.
- Refer on for specialist help where appropriate.

Training in sexuality and palliative care

All staff should receive training sessions around sexuality. The case study is a good format. The following example permits broad discussion about a variety of institutional/organisational issues: 'The hospice is about to admit a 27-year-old man with advanced rectal cancer. The admissions committee is told that he has had some surgery to change his gender and that drug treatment has given him breasts. Further surgery was cancelled subsequent to the diagnosis of cancer a year ago. The patient has a colostomy and apparently says that she prefers to be called Joan. Her next of kin is stated to be her boyfriend, Patrick. What issues might this present for the institution, the staff, the patient and her family and friends and other patients and those close to them? How should the issues be dealt with?'

Such a case example will raise issues around appropriate policies, for example admission criteria, confidentiality, a mission statement with rights of individuals and policies about the allocation of single rooms. Procedures might be those around communication from the admission group to the admitting ward and the availability of discussion groups to look at potential difficulties. For example, if the patient says that she wants to be admitted to a female bay, at what point will her rights conflict with those of other female patients to dignity and privacy? Does the unit have a policy of discussion of potentially difficult situations with the patient herself prior to admission? What procedures are in place for clinical discussion and support and education for staff? Are there adequate complaints procedures? Who needs to know what information? Will volunteers, for example, who may be involved in helping the individual to go to the toilet, be told about surgery? Any such case discussions need to be conducted without censure and always with the opportunity for staff to talk about what they really needed to ask but found it difficult to say.

Another useful format for training staff in the area of sexuality is to divide the staff into groups and present them all with a common situation. Perhaps a gay young man who is dying from AIDS is on a four-bed male bay. His partner has been lying on the bed with him in an openly physically affectionate manner. He does much to calm his dying partner. The visitors to another patient, a son and daughter, have complained to the doctor that it is unseemly for the partner to be doing this. The groups are asked to consider the feelings and concerns of the individuals involved and what they would like to say from the perspective of the patient, the partner, the doctor, the son, the daughter. These thoughts are then shared in discussion and the whole group then brainstorm what might actually help the situation.

Training must be extended to all members of staff, both paid professionals and volunteers and certainly to those involved in bereavement. We need to avoid the situation that happened in one bereavement service where a bereavement volunteer was visiting a young bereaved woman whose husband had recently died leaving her with two children. The widow said that she had long been concerned that she was a lesbian. The bereavement volunteer replied involuntarily but sharply: 'You need to think about your children. Imagine the impact of such a disclosure on them.'

Training in sexuality needs to pay particular attention to the issues of trust and safety. It must involve and challenge participants and help them feel comfortable about discussing issues about sexuality at a basic level. All sexual needs fluctuate over time and according to circumstance, our own and those of the people we care for. However, to remove 'sex' from the agenda can isolate terminally ill people even further from much needed love and acceptance when they are already facing loss in so many areas: vitality, bodily control, faith, self-confidence, control over their own destiny and energy.

We are all sexual beings and our differences should be the basis for discussion, not criticism. It is particularly encouraging to read in a booklet, *Living with Breathlessness* published by the Institute of Cancer Research, The Royal Marsden NHS Trust and Cancer Relief Macmillan Fund, a frank discussion about making love:

> Your breathlessness may make it physically very difficult for you to make love at this time, or make you apprehensive about making love in case it should cause a worsening of your breathlessness ... you can use positions that minimise breathlessness, for example you may find it easier to be in a sitting position. Avoid bending over or positions that may make you feel claustrophobic. You may find it difficult to lay underneath your partner, or you may find that standing to make love is easier ... Please feel free to talk over any difficulties you have relating to making love with any of the doctors or nurses caring for you either at home or in hospital. They will not be embarrassed and may be able to help. [Institute of Cancer Research, 1995]

The wording is frank and clear, with an open invitation that people can either pursue or leave according to their wishes.

Equally important for its firm lesson about the importance of not making assumptions was the poem given to Barbara Monroe by an elderly woman having treatment for terminal cancer. Barbara had told her that she would be absent the next day because she was going to give a group some training on sexuality. The woman came back with a poem she felt would be suitable, 'Today is not a day for adultery' by Roger McGough. It contains the wonderful verse:

> Your umbrella will leave a tell tale
> Puddle in the hall. Another stain
> To be explained away. Stay in,
> Keep your mucus to yourself.
> Today is not a day for sin.

Humour and thoughtfulness exist on both sides of the fence.

Finally, Barbara reiterates, 'Everyone needs reassurance that good sex is built on good communication, not good bodies.'

**World Health Organization Regional Office for Europe
Concepts of sexual health**

- A capacity to enjoy and control sexual and reproductive behaviour in accordance with social and personal ethic
- Freedom from fear, guilt, false beliefs and other psychological factors inhibiting sexual response and impairing sexual relationships
- Freedom from organic disorders, disease and deficiencies that interfere with sexual and reproductive functions

---

Gender and palliative care

Gender issues, for both men and women, are important in thinking about the psychosocial aspects of palliative care. Obviously there will be common concerns and features for men and women alike – death, dying and bereavement is a common human experience. At another level, however, there are specific concerns and features which many men and women will experience and process differently. Generalisations have their limitations. On the one hand, one needs to respect the commonality of experience and, on the other, the diversity. For example, 'lesbians and gay men are not a homogenous group, [they] are made up of equally diverse individuals, organisations, groups, communities and ideas' (Brown, 1997a).

In recent times, gender issues have frequently been interpreted as being synonymous with feminist issues and one must recognise the power-less position which women still experience in the structure of society. In palliative care, there are significant gender concerns in the attitude and structure of many services and daily practice issues to be confronted, for example:

- Coping in a male-dominated medical profession or a female-dominated palliative care specialty
- Is what is predominantly a counselling model in psychosocial care, operated largely by females and with women mainly as consumers, meeting the requirements of men?
- A patient with a bowel section asked, 'How will it affect me?', only to be reassured by the staff that there would be 'no problem'. What the patient was concerned about was whether he could still have anal sex
- With women predominantly having caring responsibilities, what are the implications for women employees in terms of adequate employment conditions, viz. crèche support, emergency leave, or when an employee wishes just to work the hours for which they are paid when there is an unspoken expectation that pioneering services work 'beyond the call of duty'.

Recently, there seems to be an increasing amount of research interest in palliative care, particularly in bereavement research, of the way men and women process their grief and benefit best from intervention (Bierhals et al., 1996). Schut et al. (1997) from the Centre for Bereavement Research and Intervention undertook a recent investigation of emotion-focused versus problem-focused intervention for 23 widows and 23 widowers, who were suffering elevated levels of distress eleven months after their loss. They concluded that widowers benefited more from emotion-focused intervention as men tend to focus less on their emotions and widows benefited more from problem-focused intervention as they tend to focus more on their emotions.

Clearly practice experience and qualitative research indicate ethnic and cultural variations among clients of the same gender. For example, Helen Cosis Brown, a carer interviewed in Chapter 1 comments on the contrasting behaviours between English and Welsh men in the rural setting in which her father was dying, where the Welsh males were freely and openly weeping (Brown, 1997b).

Listening to men's voices in palliative care

Malcolm Williams, Principal Social Worker, St Christopher's Hospice, London

Malcolm Williams works in a largely female setting, which is common in palliative care settings. Within the Social Work Department there are five women principal social workers: two women welfare assistants, two women administrators/secretaries and a woman director. Within the hospice, although there is an overwhelming majority of female staff, senior positions and heads of departments are occupied almost equally by males and females.

Malcolm believes that theories of grief and bereavement have to be 'genderised' – people cope differently based on biology or conditioning. Yet 'men' and 'women' cannot be completely compartmentalised: 'We often say to those who grieve that everyone must of a necessity take their own path of mourning. I believe that our past conditioning, present circumstances and our fears of the future all become part of each individual's response to loss' (Williams, 1996b).

There are variations of experiences and roles within the genders (Williams, 1996a). He has been raising the awareness of specific practices and issues around men: clients and colleagues. He realised that he was repeatedly being asked to see women within families and few husbands, partners, sons or brothers. A view or assumption was given that men do not wish to express their feelings or use talking to help them cope. Further, very limited information appeared on case records of the non-next-of-kin male members of families, making it extremely difficult to invite them to bereavement follow-up meetings or to engage them in individual or group support. They were certainly largely under-represented in bereavement follow-up.

During the phase when the patient was dying, Malcolm frequently saw men as being in the background, unless they were male spouses. Questions occurred to him: 'Who were the men involved?' 'Do they ever engage in receiving help?' 'How do we know what they are experiencing?' Women in families and as staff members seemed to act as gatekeepers to men receiving services.

Background

Malcolm's background as an experienced social worker in various fields did not allow him to concur with some of the views held. He was prompted to enquire more about the experiences of men *vis-à-vis* aspects of palliative care. He found that there is comparatively little literature directly related to men and their experience of grief and mourning. He was interested in what women writers said about men. Much of the knowledge available has been influenced by important general works on grief and bereavement. Early comment on men's experience appeared to rely on interpretation of general observation leading to what was felt to be a reasonable assumption that there may not be many essential differences in the process for men and women.

Raphael (1982), for example, remarks that patterns of normal bereavement are essentially the same for men and women but that we should always question assumptions and not make superficial judgements concerning men and women and their responses to loss. Studies have been made of spouses (Brobant, 1992; Byrne, 1996) and of men who grieve a child (Burnell, 1994; Littlewood, 1991) for example.

In entering the field of palliative care, his personal and professional experiences had led Malcolm to further question the process of managing change and in particular, how men manage change. As with other palliative care practitioners, he reflected on questions relating to people coping with change whilst living with the inevitability of death and finding ways to talk about it afterwards. How are men in particular brought up, conditioned and their life experiences constructed? Are there any common patterns?

Malcolm was keen to locate death and bereavement in their *cultural* context and this includes the place of gender. This led to further questioning of what culture demanded of men. What were the cultural expectations and prescriptions of men? What behaviour is demonstrated at a time of change such as a crisis? Malcolm's experience of men was discrepant with the myths about men not showing their feelings, not wanting to talk or wanting to be practical. He was aware, nevertheless, that men and women manage crises differently as a result of society's construction of their behaviour. Men are often perceived as not being capable of expressing emotions and vulnerability. Even in palliative care, when men show feelings and cry, there is frequently embarrassment.

Crying

With the huge emphasis in practice and in the literature on the importance of crying, and the expectation by many that men should 'have a good cry', it can be seen as a failure if men do not cry.

Practice experience has shown that some men can become irritated or angry at being pressured by professional staff or girlfriends/partners to cry. One has to also question whether women grieve better by crying more. The whole phenomenon of crying can also become a big issue in a relationship and serves to unbalance a cluster of interactions between partners and family members, for example, men being expected to continue to perform 'restoration' and organisational tasks, at the same time as entering into 'griefwork' and traditional loss behaviour (Stroebe, 1996). 'Not crying' or 'not shedding tears' may not stop the grieving process, only move grief forward in a different way.

Malcolm's speculation about men and loss and grief led him to hypothesise that men have different ways of showing grief; that they may require permission to express it; that they are under pressure to be practical, and that men remaining in control served a function of allowing others to openly grieve.

Rituals

Men have their own rituals. Malcolm's experience is that men group together and talk together, for example, at funerals. In his native Cornwall, historically, men went to funerals and women stayed at home to do the cooking; men negotiated with the funeral directors whilst women planned the services. Even in cities in modern society, families still work in an organised way with many men undertaking the more organisational tasks.

Surveys and practice questions raised

Malcolm undertook a survey of men by distributing to nursing staff 100 questionnaires. Results indicated that respondents considered that men were 'not so good' at expressing their feelings or accepting services. There was a hunch that men responded better to talking in informal settings and that female visitors often spoke on behalf of male visitors (Williams, 1997). There was some evidence that many staff were diffident about approaching men who appeared to be angry or hostile. Staff were helped by sharing ways of coping with this in practice.

A simple statistical survey was conducted of the numbers referred through the bereavement service, including their gender and their relationship to the deceased. The highest number of men referred to the bereavement service through the bereavement risk assessment form (see Chapter 6 'Bereavement care') were for male partners/spouses or sons. Subsequently a group was offered to adult sons who had experienced the loss of a parent in the previous six months. There were 36 potential group members based on reported distress at the time of death and immediately afterwards.

The experience of contacting them directly proved difficult and educational. Only four of the forms supplied clear contact information. In all other cases, Malcolm had to write a letter via a female member of the family, e.g. a mother, wife, sister. Of the number invited, ten replied and six attended the group. Significantly clearer contact information was available for male spouses/partners and for bereaved women generally. This targeting process raised a number of questions:

1. Why did we not have contact information for men other than a spouse/partner?
2. How did we introduce bereavement follow-up to male relatives/carers and was the process any different for females?
3. What were the different experiences of staff in talking with men and women about bereavement?

Another general hospice survey was conducted in 1996 using a simple questionnaire to 152 hospices in the British Isles. Information was requested about the way in which staff engaged with men in bereavement and, in particular, any organised groupwork specifically for men. Of the 66 responses, five hospices had offered gender-specific group work to men in the past year. Two of the groups were abandoned at an early stage for reasons of poor attendance. The three remaining groups offered social support and social contact for predominantly older men (over 60 years of age) (Williams, 1996a).

Informing practice

Being aware of men involved with an ill person

- Place greater emphasis on support needs of men dealing with chronic or terminal illness within their families or with partners or friends
- Encourage other family members, particularly female, to talk about the men in the family and what their experience might be
- Think about a man's significance to the ill person and enquire whether that has been acknowledged in the communication together
- Recognise that men who need support may need extra encouragement to obtain it. This may require being aware of the way family members can block access to men in the family; and the professional team acknowledging the men involved in the case to discourage possible blocking of access by staff. Be conscious of the potential difficulties posed by nearly 'all-female' environments. We can block access to men's expression if an all-female environment colludes with the view that men need to be strong and provide major supports to women. Existing theory and handed-down practice wisdom can inadvertently block honest expression of men's feelings if the way to grieve is prescribed and dogmatic.

Raising the profile on men and palliative care wherever possible in the multi-professional team, e.g. in ward rounds 'how are the sons? have they been coming in?', is important. Question generalisation and stereotyping.

Keep the topic alive and awake! For example, in preparing prayers at the hospice, Malcolm was planning to use quotations from men on what they said about their grieving.

Recording

More conscious use of the family/relationship tree to record men and observe involvement of men in the family is needed. Nursing staff should be encouraged to enter details of men in addition to details of female carers. Employ the family/relationship tree for direct discussion with significant visitors, including men.

Groupwork with staff and clients

Men's Forum for staff   a periodic meeting of any clinical male staff to discuss issues common to men in the hospice, for example, what it's like working in a female-dominated service. Some of the forum meetings have been theme-led, for example, 'Spirituality and Men'. Despite initial resistance from female staff at the idea of a meeting exclusively for men, those men who have attended have found it beneficial. The focus has been 'What's the professional perspective, but fed from the personal perspective?'

Spouses and Sons group   runs four to six sessions with six to eight members. The practitioner has to work extremely hard at getting men to come. A workshop style works better; writing is effectively used as a medium to explore feelings. Meeting earlier in the grieving process is more helpful before the men have a perception of having 'got it sorted', i.e. three to six months as opposed to six to twelve months following the bereavement.

Groups for fathers of young children are planned.

Bereavement work   scrutinises the bereavement risk assessment forms and notes the presence of the male members of families. In individual bereavement counselling, the counsellor chooses to make a firm offer to work with men and not collude with initial rejections or accept others' views that the men in the deceased's family are not interested. The bereavement volunteers have found that when men are 'given permission' to express their feelings, they do make use of the opportunities.

There are also specific support groups for bereaved men which are role-based, e.g. spouses and sons. During Bereavement Evenings, counsellors should be particularly aware of the men attending.

Some lessons learnt

- Men are not all alike, but there is some commonality of experience and coping
- Targeting men to use psychosocial services – individual and group – is difficult. A practitioner is often left reaching out to them via a female member of the family. Men are often placed in specific roles in families away from doing the 'griefwork'. Evenings and weekends are the better times to have access to men: this applies particularly to younger men with paid work commitments
- 'Men shouldn't be seen as different' denies the specific needs and requirements of the experience for many males
- Men of different status, ethnicity, sexual orientation and class process grief differently
- Men 'cry' in different ways; for example, playing snooker aggressively and then feeling better, walking, keeping active and busy: 'I'm doing all the jobs Dad wanted done and couldn't do.' (See Julie Stokes' example of the grandfather who made a memory box for his grandchildren in Chapter 3.) All the men in the groups carried photos or mementoes of the deceased. They were grieving but were not communicating this through overt emotion
- One questions the language and conventions of traditional counselling when applied to many men. For example, men talk more in informal situations such as in cars, in corridors or on landings and such communication might not be considered significant by staff if it seems too informal
- There are better practice formats to help men access services, for example, ward staff having a more pro-active role in approaching male members of families to enquire after their experiences; informal contact; ask men 'how are you grieving?'; affirm men's actual experiences rather than change their experiences; do not try to encourage men to be 'more like women'; consider what crying may mean for men under pressure to do so.

Malcolm Williams comments: 'Men should not be expected to be more like women … write down comments from men!' There is no such thing as asexual grief theory.

Resources

Albany Trust 26 Balham Hill, London SW12 9EB. Tel: 0181 767 1827
A charitable foundation to promote psychosexual health and emotional well-being through counselling, education and research

Gemma – Lesbians with/without disabilities BM Box 5700, London WC1N 3XX

Human Sexuality Unit St George's Hospital, Tooting, London SW17. Tel: 0171 672 1255

Impotence Advisory Service Freepost, Staines House, 157–172 High Street, Staines, TW18 1BR

Relate Head Office, Herbert Gray College, Little Church Street, Rugby, Warwickshire, CV21 3AP. Tel: 01788 573241

SPOD Association to Aid the Sexual and Personal Relationships of People with a Disability 286 Camden Road, London N7 0BJ. Tel: 0171 607 8851/2

Terence Higgins Trust 52–54 Gray's Inn Road, London WC1X 8JU. Tel: 0171 831 0330

Women's Therapy Centre 6–9 Manor Gardens, London N7 6LA. Tel: 0171 263 6200

6 Bereavement care

'The death of a loved one is not only a loss, it is a turning point; the world will
never be the same again. Each bereaved person faces a long period
of adjustment to a life which is seldom wanted or planned.'
(Parkes, Relf and Couldrick, 1996)

'Adaptation does not mean resolution, in the sense of some complete
'once and for all' coming to terms with the loss. Rather, it involves
finding ways to put the loss into perspective and to move on with life.'
(Walsh and McGoldrick, 1991)

Bereavement is an event; grief is the emotional response; mourning is the cultural process. Bereavement and grief are physical, spiritual, intellectual, social as well as emotional and cultural experiences. Grieving is healthy; it is not an illness. By grieving, the bereaved person adjusts to the loss: the reality of an external event is assimilated internally (Relf, 1995).

Traditionally, hospice and palliative care has continued to offer care to family, carers and friends well after the time of the death. Although bereavement work begins on the day the ill person is referred, and much of the psychosocial involvement with the family aims at preparing them for bereavement, families report that they can never be prepared enough. The moment we begin to put words to bereavement and grief and services to work with it, we risk denying the sheer uniqueness of the experience and the diversity of how the phenomena affect thinking, feeling and doing.

In hospice and palliative care, following the death, a new phase begins and a new piece of work is undertaken: 'Avoiding grief carries a price in terms of withdrawal from relationships, physical symptoms and compulsive behaviours. It is therefore essential that palliative care professionals offer at least some kind of emotional first aid to help families and individuals begin the process of mourning' (Monroe, 1993a); 'Bereavement work is invisible in the hospice/palliative care service' (Bourne, 1997).

This chapter will consider good practice in operating a bereavement service rather than focusing on counselling practice. It considers the planning, implementation, training and support involved in establishing a bereavement service in two hospices. The two services chosen are among

121

the most pioneering bereavement services in the UK: Trinity Hospice and St Christopher's Hospice have jointly almost 30 years' experience of providing care. The practitioners/managers interviewed have personally been responsible for the development and style of the bereavement services in their respective hospices.

In the early 1980s, hospice bereavement work was in its rudimentary stage. Patients were generally admitted longer as in-patients and there were fewer home care teams in existence. Public education on bereavement was less widespread as were local community bereavement services. Relatives returned to the ward and nursing staff became concerned to ensure appropriate support was given. The more formalised bereavement services began to multiply from this time following the examples of St Christopher's, Trinity and other hospices, as did information on setting up services (Earnshaw-Smith and Yorkstone, 1986; Wilkes, 1993; St Christopher's Hospice, 1994; Stroebe, Stroebe and Hansson, 1993; Payne and Relf, 1994; Stewart and Paddle, 1994; National Association of Bereavement Services, 1996; Bromberg and Higginson, 1996).

A hospice bereavement service

Sylvia Bourne, Principal Social Worker and Stephen Callus, Bereavement Services Co-ordinator, Trinity Hospice, London

Trinity Hospice is the oldest hospice in the country, with 30 beds in three wards, a large home care team serving 160 patients, a day centre and education unit. The bereavement service has been developed and is now run by the social work department of four members and a personal assistant. The day-to-day running of the bereavement service is undertaken by the bereavement services co-ordinator, a member of the team and a counsellor working with 16 volunteer counsellors. The bereavement service is part of the hospice's total response to the bereaved.

The core work of the bereavement service

The role of the bereavement service is consistent with its mission statement: 'to provide the highest achievable quality of psychological and social care of patients and those close to them'. The service aims to provide follow-up support and counselling to relatives or friends of those patients cared for by Trinity Hospice. It offers the bereaved person support and counselling either by phone or in person at the hospice or in the person's own home and usually for as long as the support or counselling is needed. 'Bereavement support' is defined as strengthening the bereaved person's coping mechanisms whilst 'bereavement counselling' offers the use of a counselling relationship to help the person look at changes she or he needs to make.

Risk assessment

A competent bereavement service will undertake careful assessment and this involves a process.

First, following the death of a patient, the nursing staff complete a four-page 'bereavement service' form, giving a picture of the bereaved relatives and others affected by the death. The bereavement service relies heavily on the nurses' awareness of bereavement need as subsequent work is fundamentally based on the nurses' initial assessment. There are clear implications for training here and effective multi-professional teamwork.

Deaths and those considered to be in need of follow-up are also discussed at weekly multi-professional ward/team meetings. The bereavement service form includes a family tree, other agencies involved and information about who was present at the time of death and what happened.

Individual or Family Risk Factors		
1. Are there children or adolescents in the immediate family? If yes, give ages:	Yes	No
2. Are there dependent family members? If yes, please specify:	Yes	No
3. Loss of constant companion/emotional support	Yes	No
4. Loss of financial provision	Yes	No
5. Loss of home feared or actual	Yes	No
6. Anxiety about making decisions	Yes	No
7. Family usually dependant, angry or clinging. If yes give details:	Yes	No
8. Family/friends unable to share feelings	Yes	No
9. Reluctance to face the illness or death	Yes	No
10. Family feel unprepared for the death	Yes	No
11. Marital or family discord. If yes, please specify:	Yes	No
12. Communication difficulties in the family	Yes	No
13. Care of patient unduly stressful	Yes	No
14. Distress over changed body image or personality	Yes	No
15. Presence of concurrent life crisis e.g. another bereavement	Yes	No

16.	Difficulty in dealing with previous losses	Yes	No
17.	History of mental illness/suicide risk. Please specify:	Yes	No
18.	Health difficulties in the family	Yes	No
19.	Lack of community support/friends	Yes	No
20.	Lack of spiritual support	Yes	No

Fig. 6.1   The bereavement service form

This form next is passed to the bereavement services co-ordinator. The bereavement services co-ordinator studies the form and aims to make an initial paper assessment of how much the bereaved person is 'at risk', i.e. are there, given our current understanding of the nature of bereavement, sufficient concern and factors present that might result in delayed or complicated grief, over-intense or extreme grief reactions, or reactions resulting in behaviour linked with bereavement?

Finally, depending on the degree of risk factors present, the co-ordinator takes one of three courses of action:

(a) To arrange for immediate or urgent contact in exceptional circumstances of need and/or risk (e.g. where there are dependent family members and a lack of community support or friends and other complicating factors such as mental illness/suicide risk). In such cases a hospice social worker is already likely to be involved and can provide time-limited intervention.

(b) To arrange for a telephone call by a bereavement counsellor to specifically offer bereavement follow-up support or counselling six to eight weeks after the death. This is offered where there are a number of risk factors in evidence, i.e. approximately 25 per cent of bereaved relatives and friends. The counsellor in telephone contact has options to offer the bereaved person: either a meeting, a further phone call or nothing other than the hospice's general invitations. On average just over half of families telephoned take up counselling contact.

(c) To send a letter with the hospice's bereavement leaflet, 'What may happen and where to find help'. This leaflet explains the general nature of grief and how the bereavement service could help. It also lists other resources and literature which bereaved people might find useful. About 70–75 per cent of those followed up by the service, where the risk or need or bereavement counselling support is felt to be low, receive a letter and leaflet.

The hospice also has available other leaflets: 'What to do when someone dies. A practical guide' and a leaflet for adults concerned for grieving children, 'Children and bereavement'.

Exceptionally there is no follow-up undertaken, e.g. where no relatives are nearby and there is limited information; or where relatives have made it clear to nursing staff that they wish to have no further contact.

Timing of follow-up

Research studies (Relf, 1989) and experience have shown that initial follow-up prior to six to eight weeks is less productive in establishing a meaningful conversation with the bereaved person who is still in the very early stages of grief. In the early weeks, the newly bereaved person is still relatively numbed and living in an 'unreal' world. As an experiment, over a three-month period, the volunteer bereavement counsellors made contact with relatives from three weeks following the death. They repeatedly found the common response was 'I'm fine!'

Responding to bereavement risk

Key factors determining whether follow-up by phone contact is imperative rather than letter follow-up are:

- Family unprepared for the death – It is common to feel unprepared but in the 'risk' context, it refers to sudden death for which relatives were especially unprepared.
- Suicide risk – Not an uncommon *feeling* to have but the threat is taken seriously and checked out if the person has gone some way beyond having a sense of life not worth living, e.g. to explore to what extent they have made any plans or taken any action that could lead to successful suicide.
- Conflict in families – Although a feature of family life, often families do manage to temporarily hold hostilities around the death bed. If there is strong hostility, overt or covert, this puts enormous additional strain at a time of emotional vulnerability.
- Excessive clinging or expression of grief – This can be quite a usual feature of grief but where there seems to be no ebbing and flowing of the grief, there can be extreme exhaustion. Sometimes people need permission to be able to put their grief aside. Such excessive expressions of grief can also indicate an overtly dependent or complicated relationship between the deceased and the bereaved.

In deciding if it is appropriate to offer bereavement follow-up or counselling, one has to ask the question, 'To what extent can the person make use of the service as offered?' Clearly someone with severe learning disabilities or a bereaved person with extreme emotional needs who may require more intensive therapy, may not be suitable for a palliative care bereavement service. It is usual that the experience of bereavement connects with and triggers all kinds of other life experiences and losses. The past is, of course, always in the present. It has to be acknowledged that there are limits to what a volunteer bereavement counselling service can offer and if there are large unresolved issues from the past, then other forms of counselling or therapy could be more appropriate.

Recruitment, selection, training and supervision of bereavement counsellors

The hospice's 16 volunteer bereavement counsellors come from a range of backgrounds, e.g. therapists, counsellors, trainee counsellors on placement or people who have had experience of bereavement.

The selection process is a careful one with open meetings for potential applicants, individual interviews before the course and formal selection interviews after the course. The formal selection interview is held with two interviewers, one from the bereavement and social work team and the other from another department of the hospice.

Training has comprised two terms of the bereavement unit of the diploma in palliative care held at Trinity (115 hours), ward experience (12 hours) and a foundation course on self-awareness and counselling skills (26 hours). Prospective counsellors pay for their training initially but 60 per cent of their fee is reimbursed if they are accepted by Trinity. A new style of integrated course is to commence offering two terms' training, over 80 hours. Ward experience is no longer obligatory; instead issues of dying are included in the course and hospice induction sessions are offered to counsellors following selection.

Continuing training comprises a series of one day or evening workshops and attendance at outside courses. Each new volunteer is asked to sign a volunteer agreement agreeing to abide by their job description, code of practice for volunteers, health and safety and equal opportunities policies.

The counsellor's role straddles both counselling and support. The bulk of their work takes place within the first three to six months of bereavement with an average of six sessions provided. Counsellors have between two and seven clients. Over half of the counselling sessions take place in the hospice. Forty per cent of cases are closed (by agreement) after three months' work. If counselling continues for one year, the contract with the bereaved person is carefully reviewed. The counselling must have a bereavement content or other more general counselling might be more appropriate. Also, the hospice is very clear that it aims to help people to move on in their grief, not to encourage long-term support.

Counsellors complete forms to report on their initial assessment, review, closing and a monthly statistical return. They are also encouraged to complete review and closing forms with their client. Attendance at fortnightly supervision sessions as part of one of three small supervision groups is the heart of the bereavement service. Individual additional supervision is provided for new counsellors or those with particularly difficult caseloads. All counsellors have one review/appraisal session each year.

Trinity Hospice

Job Description for a Volunteer Bereavement Counsellor

Role

Your role is to provide follow-up support and counselling to the bereaved families and others close to patients who have died in the care of Trinity Hospice. It includes:

- carrying a minimum caseload of two clients
- attending a fortnightly counselling supervision group at the hospice, at least 18 times in any one year
- attending one of the evenings for remembering at least once a year.

You are accountable to the bereavement services co-ordinator.

Commitment

- The commitment to the hospice bereavement service is for two years after initial training and formal interview
- The first four months will be a probationary period with a review at the end of this period.

Our responsibilities to you

You can expect the hospice bereavement service:

- to value your enthusiasm, willingness, expertise and potential
- to train you to an appropriate level
- to support you with on-going supervision and training
- to respect your needs and limitations.

This includes taking time out from working as a bereavement counsellor to attend to your other needs or to take a rest, and your right to decline a client or ask for a client to be re-referred to another counsellor.

- to provide you, once yearly, with an opportunity to review and appraise your work as a hospice bereavement counsellor
- to pass on to you any relevant communications from clients quickly
- to provide reasonable access to the coordinator or your supervisor including being able to contact them at home
- to provide you with timely information about hospice events which might involve you as a bereavement counsellor.

Additionally you can also expect the hospice:
- to provide adequate insurance cover
- to provide adequate rooms for counselling and supervision to take place
- to reimburse you for any reasonable expense incurred in relation to your work as a volunteer.

This includes postage, telephone costs and any travelling to clients' homes or the hospice, including travel to supervision and further training.

Your responsibilities to us
- a commitment to your own on-going development as a volunteer bereavement counsellor
- to attend group supervision as stated above
- that you respect confidentiality in relation to your volunteer bereavement work.

The co-ordinator must be informed of and agree to any supervision you may receive outside the hospice bereavement service for your work as a hospice bereavement counsellor.

- to disclose to your supervisor the fact of any gift being made to you by a client, and to direct a client desiring to make a monetary gift to send that gift to the hospice directly

  You are free to keep a gift that is small, consumable or perishable.
- to take a sabbatical from working as a volunteer bereavement counsellor, usually for at least a year, where you have experienced a significant personal loss

  This would usually involve making alternative arrangements for the client caseload you are carrying at that time.
- that where you keep personal records of your work with clients that these are kept *confidentially* and that you agree to destroy any such notes and records when counselling with a particular client ceases, unless the agreement of the co-ordinator or supervisor is obtained
- to complete and submit in good time, any assessment, review or closing forms for each client, including a monthly record of client contacts
- to contribute to any evaluation, audit or research that may from time to time be intended to help improve the services offered
- to abide by the hospice's code of practice for volunteers.

'Evening for remembering'

About one year after the death, relatives and friends are invited to an evening service to remember the person who has died. The events take the format of either a Christian service or a non-religious format and families have the choice of which they attend. The service ends with refreshments and informal discussion. The bereavement counsellors attend in order to provide informal support. About 25 per cent of families of patients who died at Trinity attend and as a result of attendance, some participants have asked for longer-term counselling support.

Painting project

The innovation has been a 'painting special memories' project. Building on the therapeutic quality of painting, one of the bereavement counsellors, an artist herself, has been working individually with bereaved relatives to paint for them their special memories. With greater awareness of the place of memories and biography in the bereavement process, there is great potential value in this media and the process it evokes (Walter, 1996). The project is pioneering and has been funded by the Omega Foundation, a charity that supports art in palliative care.

The medium of painting is used along with the bereavement counsellor's talking and listening skills to produce a concrete outcome as a result of the work in which she is engaged with the client. The work takes between two and four sessions with the artist/counsellor producing a water colour. Hitherto 17 clients have entered this initial project which has been evaluated. Plans are underway to initiate a larger project.

Anniversary card

A card is sent to families to arrive on the first anniversary of the death. The card is of a natural scene and is hand-written by a volunteer. The feedback indicates that people do appreciate the cards.

Audit

Trinity Hospice looks to bereavement research, good practice and audit to inform its work and is currently developing written standards of practice: 'I have found that people often erroneously interchange such terms as data collection, evaluation, research and audit. You can only audit a written measurable standard. However, evaluation, for example, may be part of the process of producing your standard. Used appropriately, audit can be another way of listening to client need' (Sylvia Bourne).

In addition, feedback from the audit will inform any changes to the service provided, and may require alterations to the written standard, which will, in turn, be audited, and thus the cycle continues.

Trinity Hospice

Bereavement Service: draft standards

Standard one
All of those contacts assessed as being at risk to be contacted on an individual basis by a member of the bereavement services team by phone or letter within eight weeks of the date of death of the patient. Target: 85%

Standard two
All contacts which have been assessed as at risk are then assessed as either being urgent or non-urgent. Those contacts assessed as being urgent are contacted within six weeks of the date of death of the patient rather than eight weeks.   Target: 100%

Standard three
All of those clients assessed as needing to be referred to another agency are given the appropriate information to enable them to make contact.   Target: 100%

Standard four
All counsellors to have an average minimum of one counselling or supervision contact each week (unless there are special circumstances such as time away or illness).   Target: 100%

Standard five
All counsellors to attend a minimum of 18 of the 26 group supervisions and two individual supervisions scheduled between 1 April ... and 31 March ... Students on placement needing to meet British Association for Counselling supervision requirements should attend a minimum of one hour's supervision for eight hours' client contact time during the period of their placement.   Target: 100%

Standard six
All counsellors to have satisfactorily completed the Trinity Hospice counselling training or an equivalent training and spent a minimum of six volunteer sessions on a ward in Trinity Hospice.   Target: 100%

Standard seven
All volunteer counsellors to commit to a minimum of 18 months as volunteer bereavement counsellors.   Target: 100%

Standard eight
All counsellors to have signed a working agreement with Trinity Hospice bereavement service and to have a copy of the agreement. (NB The agreement is currently being drafted.)   Target: 100%
Auditing
Standards 1, 2 and 3 to be monitored and audited every three months
Standards 4 and 5 to be monitored and audited every six months
Standards, 6, 7 and 8 to be monitored and audited every twelve months

Current plans

Plans to offer group work for adult bereaved children and to further develop bereavement work with children, adolescents and their families is actively being planned. Presently there is only one counsellor from minority ethnic groups (an Indian counsellor) despite the multi-ethnic nature of the area – there are plans to recruit further counsellors from minority ethnic communities.

A conversation with Barbara Monroe on team practice in bereavement

Barbara Monroe, Director of Social Work, St Christopher's Hospice, London

St Christopher's Hospice has a large well-established social work department which runs the bereavement service. The department comprises a director and six experienced social workers, a welfare assistant and a personal assistant who conducts the administration of the bereavement service. There are 25 bereavement visitors, selected by the social work department and given a free, four-month training course.

What do you aim to provide with the bereavement service?

We try to provide a service that is as appropriate as possible to the needs that are expressed both by the bereaved families and professional carers, bearing in mind that the service needs to be realistic in terms of our personnel and financial resources. We attempt to minimise the number of families needing input after the death by providing as much help as possible before the death. The end result of my period at St Christopher's is a real belief that it is possible to do some preventive work in the support you give families before, by giving information about the illness and the likely progress towards death, about the kinds of feelings they could experience, giving them a shape into which they can pour their unformed feelings and giving them some idea as to how things might be. With somebody who is finding it difficult sitting with a relative who is dying, we suggest a way they might do that, and do it with them, for example, saying 'you might like to hold their hand', while making sure that we understand what people's fears are that may prevent them from doing the things they would like to have been able to have done while the person's alive. Or indeed we find out what their lack of resources are – personal or otherwise. We make sure we know whether people would like to be there … and let them know that that might not be possible. It is important to *rehearse* different possibilities. These are the sorts of ways one can help people think about the things they wish to say or do before the death. We need to make sure our professionalism does not exclude families who may or may not wish to join in with practical caring tasks. Information given in advance can sometimes help to prevent later misunderstandings, e.g. that a change from oral medication to injections may become necessary and why very ill people eat and drink less and less.

It is interesting that we target as 'at risk,' and have a higher take-up of help (one-third more), from families whose relative has been a patient for less than 48 hours.

We give information on feelings they might anticipate – especially where children are concerned – so they are not too shocked when it arrives.

Immediately after the death

There is another set of good bereavement practices that concern managing the time immediately after the death (the hour or two after and then the first day or two), and can help make the experience of bereavement somewhat more manageable. Sometimes you have to be quite active in managing this period of time. If there is a family in conflict or if one or two members are having difficulty in retaining any kind of emotional control, you can do a lot to prevent bad memories later on of what happened, by being quite active, on other people's behalf. I remember a man who died of a bleed, quite unexpectedly, when his wife just arrived to take him home. She was quite insistent that she still take him home, although she was covered in blood. Some staff felt she should be taken elsewhere to be calmed down.

What she needed was for somebody to be with her, with him. By being involved in washing him, she gradually calmed down and slowly began to process the experience. She later spoke very movingly of how important an experience it was of having washed him and of laying him out and that that became the more powerful memory.

In another situation, a man who had physically abused all his children and sexually abused his daughters over many years was dying in the hospice. The children were having great difficulty coming to see him. They were now adults and there were complex negotiations between the hospice staff and the family about whether they wished to see him or not. One daughter came to see him. He wanted them to be there but could not ask for forgiveness or admit to the things that had happened.

After the death, a son came to view the body and picked up a comb and began to comb his father's hair. That piece of contact was so important in securing some kind of reconciliation that he had not been able to make in person verbally during the father's illness.

If we can be very aware and sensitive at these times, there are some quite small symbolic things that can be very large and powerful in people's later memories.

Sometimes our practice is about managing ourselves and our colleagues' responses at this time. One has to stave off the sense of panic and crisis long enough. As a practitioner, there is no set way of knowing what to do. One just has to be alert to what is happening in the situation and to opportunities for making suggestions. You need to be confident enough to know that the situation will unwrap itself in some way that will be positive and, at worst, you will have at least held people for long enough for the family to gather itself. A lot of what I do is just 'spinning it out', putting words around unfamiliar situations in order for people not to have to process things too fast.

The same is helpful when people come to view the body and receive the death certificate. Very often people are 'galloping' and part of our practice is to find a mechanism to 'slow them down'. In addition, one thinks of and gives little prompts about the areas they might wish to mention, ask about, to share.

Part of our role is giving family members, immediately after the death, reminders about who they think would like to be present, who do they need to let know, while at the same time letting them know that they do not have to let others know. Sometimes an advocacy role is undertaken as other family members wish to make decisions for a newly bereaved relative, e.g. whether the relative returns home to sleep in the double bed or if they go to another relative's house. One tries to ensure that grieving relatives do what they feel they want to do and is right for them as an individual and as a family. Cultural considerations are, of course, essential at this point.

Relatives are told that there will be opportunities to talk about practical aspects the next day. At this moment in time, people just need to be the relationship they are. The early experiences and feelings are very important and can so easily become lost if they are side-tracked by practical considerations.

At home it is a little different, but the home care team would have discussed in advance the actions, if possible, that would be necessary to take in terms of removal of the body and funeral directors. Again the aim is to give people choices and to try and remove some of the paralysis engendered by fear of the unknown: to discuss, for example, whether the parents will wake children up if the death happens in the middle of the night.

The family are told that the meeting the next day is open to anyone who would like to attend and often children are involved.

The day after death

Helping people begin to grieve

Practice within the in-patient unit has a structured format and involves telling the family that we are going to be giving them the death certificate and that the staff will be returning belongings to them. They are also told that they will have an opportunity of asking any questions about the illness and the death itself.

Concern is expressed as to how relatives are feeling and early on in the session, family members are alerted to the fact that they will have the choice of seeing the body and that they do not have to decide yet. The importance of warning is underlined and that people should not be forced to make a decision about viewing the body as they arrive. They need time to settle down. It is acknowledged that in some busy hospital situations, it is not always possible to manage the logistics of viewing times as one would wish.

Opportunity to ask questions

A catalytic question is sometimes, 'Although I know you knew he/she was going to die, I am wondering if things moved quite fast in the end and perhaps there are bits you'd like to go over again?' One tries to communicate that it is all right 'to have muddles' whilst still trying to slow down the activity. People cannot begin to process what has happened if they cannot begin to understand the facts or if they have a question mark over an issue. Let people know that questions are OK.

Death certificate and information

Giving the death certificate is an ideal opportunity of exploring queries and questions. Allowing relatives to take time to look at the death certificate, to clarify the cause of death and uncertainties about diagnosis is important.

At this point, leaflets about 'What to do after a death' from the Department of Social Security are given. Details are provided about registering the death and exact location of the registrar is clarified. Clear information is provided verbally and written down, remembering that it can be very hard to process information when newly bereaved.

Letting people know there are choices

Plans and ideas for the funeral are checked out in terms of any preferences the deceased expressed, not to take over from the role of family members and friends, but rather to remind people that there are choices that can be made. Often people have never been to a funeral before and they are given a chance to think about burial or cremation, the type of service, costs, etc. It is important to quietly let them know that they do not have to accept set ways of doing funerals or other people's choices. So often bereaved relatives in bereavement groups will express distress that they did not have more of a say in the funeral arrangements.

Opportunity to see the body

Once relatives are a little more relaxed, they are invited to view the body: 'I am wondering how you feel about going to see —?' The very personalised nature of the decision to view or not is made clear and that it is not a requirement. They are asked if they have viewed a dead person before and told that a member of staff will be with them. The viewing arrangements are explained in detail so people know what to expect. Preparation is important. It is emphasised that they can all make a different choice and that nobody need be alone because a member of staff will join them if they wish.

Once at the viewing room, relatives are offered a choice as to whether they wish to remain alone or not, allowing choice but with little prompts (e.g. 'you can take as long as you like' and modelling that touching and stroking is acceptable if they wish to).

Bereavement leaflet.

During this meeting, leaflets are given to relatives on the nature of bereavement and as many copies are provided as necessary for other friends and family members. Everyone is made aware that they are welcome to contact the service for counselling or advice. The bereavement service is offered pro-actively to anyone identified as being at risk and to anyone who asks for it.

Part of the challenge as a practitioner in helping people who are in psychological crisis following the death and who are emotionally labile, is that one is attempting to find the appropriate combination between 'managing' and taking charge of the situation, whilst responding to the unique and changing reactions of the bereaved person.

One of the tasks of the team following the death is to demystify the experience of death and dying and to make it manageable. Involvement can create positive memories for surviving relatives and, as practitioners, we have to break down these tasks into manageable proportions. Without denying the experience of the bereaved people themselves, it is useful to communicate that, as practitioners, 'we have had the benefit of being with a number of families at this time of their lives and we know that often what people find beneficial is —.' It is important to emphasise, for example, that grief is different for everyone and each individual in the family will find their own way and time, so they need to be gentle with each other.

Part of our work in empowering and freeing people is getting them to a point where they can know that there is the possibility of a choice, without pressing them to choose. If people want to vacillate or sit on the fence, that is their choice. This applies throughout palliative care over issues related to talking openly about the illness and death or during bereavement.

Rehearsal

One technique one uses in palliative care generally and during bereavement in particular, is the idea of rehearsal. It is important to help families predict situations: 'Is there anybody you might find difficult to tell about what's happened?' 'How do you think you might do that?' 'What might happen?' 'Is there a way of doing it so that doesn't happen?' 'Who are you worried about?' This is part of the process of opening up possibilities for people and giving them some sense of control. How they move into those possibilities or not is then up to them.

This is skilled and subtle work and when watching a practitioner doing it well, the 'work' is almost imperceptible; it looks like conversation – the words are ordinary. These are moments when you use some small interventions to respect people's individuality and to show your understanding of how much they are hurting.

Expressing appreciation

It is important to find a way of acknowledging the family's care of the dead person – they need to know they have done a good job. It is not uncommon for staff to hear, for example, during the time of bereavement support, 'The nurse said we did well to have kept him at home.'

As staff, if we share a personal memory, it encourages the bereaved family to begin to express their own memories. Letting people say 'thank you' and 'goodbye' to staff, in their own way, and not cutting this process short, can be helpful to newly bereaved families. These expressions are part of the process of the families' separation from the professionals and of re-establishing their independence and integrity.

Bereavement risk assessment forms

During the course of the illness, the nursing staff record information about both facts and concerns about family members who might be at risk in bereavement. For example, if they become aware that a family member had, in fact, a depressive illness or psychiatric treatment, they would record that fact.

The form on which this information is recorded is fully completed within 24 hours of the 'day after the death' meeting. This includes information about events at the point of death and the subsequent meeting. Opinions are expressed about possibly significant occurrences and relationships, such as an ambivalent relationship with the deceased. The family or relationship tree is included on the form.

The forms are an important snapshot of the family and indicate a likelihood of emotional and psychological risk in bereavement. They are valuable for the nurses in terms of letting go of the piece of work and reassuring in that they have conveyed their concerns regarding family and friends to another arm of the service.

The forms are analysed by the social work department and a decision is made as to whether bereavement is offered pro-actively or not. There is no weighting on the form or points indicating level of risk. As mentioned in the bereavement leaflet, there is an open invitation to all to use the bereavement service.

Where there is concern, contact is made eight to ten weeks following the death. St Christopher's offers help to about one quarter of bereaved families. Experience has shown that there is a greater take-up of service then than after four weeks. At this stage, the bereavement volunteers make a firm move to visit rather than an open offer: 'I would like to come and see you.' The aim is to make an assessment visit, as the very factors that have targeted somebody as being at risk may mean that they find it difficult to request help for themselves.

Very occasionally there is a need for immediate bereavement work, e.g. where there are no other relatives or friends, or an overt suicide risk.

After three months

Every bereaved family is invited by letter to a bereavement evening three months after the death. The evening is a one-off invitation. Transport and baby-sitting are offered and anyone from 15 years of age and above is welcome. The invitation contains another offer to contact the hospice for individual help.

Bereavement evenings

Sixty to seventy bereaved people attend a bereavement evening. Drinks are served followed by a talk given by a member of the social work department, although staff from all the different professions at the hospice are present together with bereavement volunteers.

Staff are introduced and the bereaved people told that they will have an opportunity to talk to individual team members at the end of the evening. The talk on bereavement sets the scene and people are prepared for a small group discussion.

Name labels are given to members of the groups and families are split up. Groups of ten, including two facilitators, meet for an hour. At the end of the evening, groups meet together again, members can ask questions of individual staff and the evening ends with a non-denominational moment of remembrance, taken by a chaplain.

Reminders are given of the availability of the bereavement service at the hospice. The bereavement evenings are deliberately one-off in order to avoid long-term dependence and to help people move on in their bereavement. If bereaved people need more social clubs and contact, each bereavement volunteer is furnished with an up-to-date list of local resources, e.g. University of the Third Age, gardening clubs, etc.

Individual work with a bereavement visitor

Each bereaved client receives written material about the service underlining confidentiality but also indicating that the bereavement volunteer is supervised by a member of the social work department.

All bereavement volunteers make a contract with the client, commonly for three or four sessions, subject to mutual renewal. Six to eight visits is the most common pattern, although the work can continue until after the first anniversary of the death. The contract acts as a safeguard to clients being able to end contact with a bereavement volunteer, particularly if the client was not comfortable and did not feel able to express this. Contract-making is also sound therapeutically and focuses the work.

For particularly complex or at-risk situations, the social work department and bereavement volunteer have access to the hospice's consultant psychiatrist, Dr Colin Murray Parkes, for consultation. He can see a client jointly with a bereavement volunteer.

The supervision of the bereavement volunteers is undertaken individually once a month by a social worker. They also have group case consultation sessions twice monthly.

The social workers carry a small caseload of complex cases, e.g. where there are at-risk children in a family.

Groups

Bereavement volunteers co-lead groups with the social workers, for bereaved people with common needs, e.g. children, adolescents, partners, men, etc. They are usually short-term, 'closed' groups. (See Chapter 4 'Working with groups'.)

Children and families

The social work department has produced two booklets, 'Someone special has died' for younger children and 'Your parent has died' for teenagers. Work with individual bereaved children and their families is undertaken by some of the bereavement volunteers and by social workers, although it is recognised that working with parents and children prior to the death gives many families themselves the confidence and resources they need to meet the challenge of bereavement. (See Chapter 3 'Working with families'.)

The anniversary

If the bereavement volunteer is in touch at the time of the first anniversary of the death, contact is not terminated then, but a final contact would be made after the anniversary date. For many, the anniversary is a painful time after which people often move on in their grief. For others, the second year is particularly painful.

Thanksgiving services are held throughout the year and are co-ordinated by the chaplaincy department for relatives and friends about a year after the death.

Anniversary cards are sent to all next of kin of a deceased patient but their value needs to be clarified. Very occasionally there are complaints where 'bereaved' people have moved on in the sense of having begun another relationship and they do not wish to be reminded.

Endings

Bereavement volunteers are encouraged to share their recording with clients to reinforce progress that has been made, e.g. 'This is where you were and this where you are now.' It is essential that we say goodbye to families and help them move on in their lives.

Bereavement – the whole team's concern

It is essential to attempt to integrate the bereavement service with the total palliative service, so it does not become the exclusive property of those running it – shared ownership is part of its success. At St Christopher's Hospice this is done in a number of ways:

- The multi-professional induction has three sessions on the work of the social work department including working with families; the impact of illness and death on families, and what is bereavement? This is attended by all staff in the first two weeks' employment
- All nursing staff have two further training sessions on the bereavement risk assessment form and the day after death meeting/bereavement follow-up visit for home care
- All staff who attend the bereavement evening, also attend a training session on group facilitation, gaining valuable group work skills
- All nurses and doctors attend one bereavement volunteers' group consultation session as observers
- Those staff who attend the bereavement evenings appreciate the skills of the bereavement volunteers.

Recruitment of bereavement volunteers

There are a number of factors when considering the recruitment of bereavement volunteers:

- Advertising – Try the local and minority press, e.g. *The Voice*, libraries, trade unions, Citizens Advice Bureaux, personal letters to minority ethnic groups
- Criteria – There are no specific requirements for counselling qualifications or previous educational requirements in order to attract bereavement visitors from a wide range of the community. Some trainees will require additional support, e.g. the builder for whom many of the theoretical concepts about bereavement were totally new. All trainees are offered the opportunity to see an individual tutor outside the group sessions
- Training – Volunteers' training consists of 18 weekly sessions of two-and-a-half hours. Emphasis is placed on training about race awareness and culture. All established bereavement volunteers also receive an ongoing training session once a month
- Support – There are plans to link new bereavement volunteers during their probationary period with experienced bereavement volunteers.

Lessons learned for practice

Work with newly and acutely bereaved relatives and friends involves the whole range of good communication and interpersonal skills. Predicting questions, warning and rehearsing, comfortable pacing and opening up choices are all helpful approaches. Multi-professional teamwork is the key.

Running a palliative care bereavement service, with generally a very large turnover of deaths, requires substantial organisation and attention to detail, in processing contacts with relatives, assessment processes, and in the selection, training and support of volunteers, if used. We believe that bereavement is a natural phenomenon, and with good preparation and support for family members prior to the death, the majority will cope with bereavement with their usual support networks. A bereavement service will be in touch with the more needy people. A range of skills is required beyond pure counselling skills as, on occasion, the hospice is working with some very vulnerable people psychologically, in disturbed and disturbing circumstances, with the suicidal and young children, and with adolescents and their families. Mental health training and ability to work with GPs and other community-based colleagues are required.

A palliative care bereavement service is not now a cheap option as our knowledge of bereavement has increased and expectations of quality of service have risen.

It would seem that the specific role for a palliative care bereavement service, although determined by other resources in the area, would commonly have aims related to:

1. To 'normalise' grief
2. To promote healthy grieving
3. To provide support to those in special need and those 'at risk'
4. To provide or refer for more specialist help those who are stuck or whose grieving is complicated.

These aims are realised through supportive links and information (leaflets on bereavement, follow-up phone calls and letters); good assessment and risk prediction (identification of bereavement risk factors, review); and structured opportunities to promote grieving and to invite families to seek help (support and counselling, groups, remembrance events, anniversary cards).

Key components for a successful bereavement service	
1. Management support	*Principles:* Bereavement work = risk work. It needs to be 'owned' by the service. Implications for staff need to be considered: budgets, complaints, angry clients, risk-taking.

	Practice: Is management support built into mission statement? Is it one of the service's priorities? Is it integrated with the entire service.
2. Staff	Co-ordinator of administrative and therapeutic expertise. Broad skill-mix: attention to detail; experience of working with families; multi-professional experience. Consider advantages and disadvantages of a co-ordinator not involved with the family work before the death. Administrative input essential.
3. Assessment procedures	Multi-professional decisions on criteria for specific follow-up. Training for colleagues operating procedures (e.g. administrative and nursing staff).
4. Printed material	Agree common parts of service, e.g. bereavement leaflet, letter offering support, invitation to groups, remembrance services, anniversary cards.
5. Recruitment/selection/ training/development/ support/supervision	Agree support system and outside consultation of bereavement visitors *or* professional employed staff. Counsellors, psychologists and social workers can undertake the bereavement follow-up but it is time-consuming and realistic staffing hours are required.

Resources

Bereavement Research Forum Sir Michael Sobell House, Churchill Hospital, Oxford, OX3 7LJ. Tel: 01865 225878

Compassionate Friends 53 North Street, Bristol, BS3 1EN. Tel: 0117 966 5202 Helpline: 0117 953 9639

Child Death Helpline Bereavement Services Department, Great Ormond Street Hospital NHS Trust, Great Ormond Street, London WC1N 3JH. Tel: 0171 813 8551 Helpline: 0800 282986

Cruse Bereavement Care Cruse House, 126 Sheen Road, Richmond, Surrey TW9 1UR. Tel: 0181 940 4818/9047

Jewish Bereavement Counselling Service PO Box 6748, London N3 3BX. Tel: 0181 349 0839

Lesbian and Gay Bereavement Project Vaughan M. Williams Centre, Colindale Hospital, London NW9 5HG. Tel: 0181 200 0511 Helpline: 0181 455 8894

National Association of Bereavement Services 20 Norton Folgate, Bishopsgate, London E1 6DB. Tel: 0171 247 0617

7 Achieving accessible and appropriate services

'Good care begins when difference is recognised.'
(Frank, 1991)

Whilst recognising that *everyone* is entitled to access hospice and palliative care services and that these should be appropriate to meet individual needs, it is also recognised that health care services have traditionally found it difficult to respond to the needs of some individuals or groups in society. It is generally accepted that certain groups and individuals are denied equal opportunities and experience discrimination. Ethnic, racial, religious and national minorities, lesbians and gay men, people with physical and learning disabilities and infirmity of old age are among those who require specific provision to obtain services at the same level of acceptability as those in the mainstream and without diminishing the quality of service to the majority. Within any health specialism, attempts would be made to provide for a patient with an unusual or uncommon condition. The same principles should apply to those who have particular requirements as a result of their culture or life style.

However, there are also the less visible groupings in society, with less ability to voice their needs, e.g. the very poor, the profoundly deaf, the poorly educated, certain social classes, those with less endearing personalities. In many ways people who are chronically and terminally ill are amongst the most disempowered groups in the community, particularly if they have no articulate carers, as day-to-day survival is the priority; frequently time is short and the immediate demands of the illness take over leaving little time or opportunity to advocate one's needs. Ill people and their carers come from all sections and walks of life. Their inevitable anxiety and discomfort will be exacerbated if in addition to illness, they are also alienated by professionals or services as a result of being perceived to be different in some way.

In practice, how often have we been subject to a colleague whose reaction to people is 'he's a typical —' and is prepared to 'box' patients and families into categories so that subsequent behaviour is interpreted through the lens of the stereotype? In a specialty that has grown up around identifying the individuality and changing preferences of the people it serves, the challenge appears to be about balancing the common needs and requirements of the groups to which the patient and family belong, whilst recognising the unique characteristics and traits of individuals. A practitioner must remind herself that 'everybody is different' while acknowledging that, alongside that difference, there are specific and common requirements, a certain commonality of experience that has to be taken into account.

Culture and ethnicity

One area that highlights many of the points pertinent to issues around 'working with difference' and those with minority features, is in working with people from a different culture or ethnicity from your own: 'There is a widespread feeling in the British palliative care community that people from minority ethnic populations are under-represented among the users of services for the dying. Unfortunately, few systematic data are available' (Smaje and Field, 1997).

Research suggests that generally black* and minority ethnic groups in Britain have unequal access and that their health experiences are worse than those of other groups (Haroon-Iqbal, 1995). The minority ethnic population constitutes approximately six per cent of the UK population. Sixty per cent of the black population and 36 per cent of the Asian population reside in the greater London area in the south-east with Leicester and Birmingham having the next highest percentage (National Council, 1995b).

It is primarily in these areas that issues concerning the promotion of opportunities for minority groups to access services and of adapting these services to meet needs appropriately will be of greatest concern; however, people from minority ethnic and other groups live all over the UK and require suitable provision.

The National Health Service and Community Care Act 1990, which has so much influenced the face of health and social services provision at the turn of this century, clearly supported the need to develop an ethnically–sensitive approach to community care: 'The Government recognises that people from different cultural backgrounds may have particular needs and problems ... Good community care will take account of the circumstances of minority communities and will be planned in consultation with them' (Department of

---

* The terms 'black' and 'Asian' are used in the 1991 Census with 'black' referring to 'Black Caribbean', 'Black African' or 'Black Other' groups. 'Asian' refers to 'Indian'. 'Pakistani' or 'Bangladeshi' groups.

Health, 1989). This has been promoted by the Patient's Charter: 'Respect for privacy, dignity and religious and cultural beliefs' (Department of Health, 1991). The Charter standard is that all health services should make provision so that proper personal consideration is shown.

Opening doors

A small but significant piece of research for palliative care published in 1995 by the National Council for Hospice and Specialist Palliative Care Services demonstrated that hospice and palliative care services are being used by some people from minority ethnic communities and will be increasingly needed as the proportion of the black and Asian population aged 55 and over will grow significantly over the next decade.

The findings identified the need for hospice and palliative care services to provide culturally sensitive services in respect of *language, religion, spiritual* and *dietary needs* and for particular attention to be given to providing *appropriate* and *accessible information* to these communities. The findings also showed that although hospices have done much to meet the differing needs of their patients from these minorities, it is evident that policies and systems need to be put in place to meet future requirements, e.g. *ethnic monitoring* and more consistent *referral arrangements* from general practitioners and hospitals. In addition, *staff training* and *information* is necessary in meeting the care needs of black and minority ethnic patients.

Other studies have concluded that providers of palliative care need to examine their policy and practice with regard to whether they are acceptable, accessible and culturally sensitive (Haroon-Iqbal, 1995).

Practitioners in palliative care are vigilant to provide, wherever possible, total care. The holistic nature of pain is assessed. 'Cultural pain' exists and in its widest definition colours all the other pain – physical, social, spiritual, financial and psychological.

This chapter will focus on three contrasting hospice and palliative care units which have confronted accessible and appropriate service in very different ways to meet identified needs in the communities they serve. They are all good examples of what can be achieved with some careful planning. The Acorns Children's Hospice provides a service to children and families within Birmingham, which has a very high concentration of Asian families; the North London Hospice aims to meet the needs of communities of different religious faiths, and London Lighthouse works with those who are HIV positive.

The work described in this chapter links with four areas of practice; these are known as equality of opportunity, anti-discrimination, 'working with difference' and specifically work with different cultural, ethnic and religious groups.

Acorns Children's Hospice, Birmingham

Hardev Notta, Asian Link Officer and Brian Warr, Director of Care Services

Acorns Children's Hospice is an independent hospice. It comprises a ten-bed purpose-built unit offering six respite and four emergency or terminal care beds to children and young people under the age of 19, with progressive and terminal conditions. Included in its facilities are a hydrotherapy pool and a multi-sensory room.

Four main teams provide a comprehensive service: the in-house team; the activities team providing teaching and education; the volunteer team offering direct work with children (befriending, play, home support); and the community team of 14 members covering the West Midlands Health Authority area. The multi-professional team of counsellors, nurses, occupational therapists, social workers, teachers and youth workers also include one Asian Link Officer and one Bereavement Officer for black and ethnic minority groups.

The geographical area served by the hospice includes an approximately 25 per cent South Asian (Indian, Sri Lankan, Pakistani and Bangladeshi) community and African-Caribbean population. The proportion of minority ethnic community families being helped by the hospice was representative of those of the general population of the area, a tremendous achievement. For example, of the 202 ill children currently on the hospice caseload and the 100 receiving bereavement care 30 per cent are of South Asian origin.

When many other hospice and palliative care services are finding it difficult to attract referrals from minority ethnic groups, despite sometimes substantial numbers in the population, how has this been achieved?

Acorns has a comprehensive approach to ensuring their service is accessible and appropriate. This is based on a multi-faceted look at provision where issues of access for all and meeting specific needs of minority ethnic groups permeate all aspects of the hospice service: staff, management, policy, environment, communication, community development, religion, customs and rituals and training.

Community development

A considerable investment of time and energy has 'won over' the minority ethnic communities and ensured active support and a full understanding of the service. A series of visits to groups, clubs and community leaders provided an opportunity not only to tell them about Acorns but also to ask them for their views and concerns and suggestions. This exchange and feedback from the groups has been characteristic of how staff at Acorns have worked.

A video of Acorns (paid for by an Asian businessman), translated into six community languages, and including invitations to visit the hospice, consolidated the developing relationship with the communities. The importance of responding reassuringly to concerns regarding, for example, boys being nursed by males and girls being nursed by females and clarifications about the freedom to bring personal items (e.g. own bedding) into the hospice, is underlined.

Providing information and establishing two-way communication appears to have been a crucial part in the building of trust and confidence in the sincerity of the service. Respecting the oral tradition of the cultures concerned, numerous talks were given to community groups of all sizes and in religious and non-religious venues. Through this period of community development, the word spread by word of mouth that Acorns was a place where children would be safe and comfortable and where families would be respected.

Staff

Management

An ethos within Acorns where management support and respect the need for accessible and appropriate services set an expectation of certain standards and behaviour for staff to follow. Managers within the hospice convey that they are actively committed to the message of respect for minority ethnic groups through the statements and policies developed (e.g. Equal Opportunities Policy), the active support for developments seen as necessary by the Asian Link Officer and user groups (e.g. Women's Group), and the emphasis given to feedback from individual users.

Specialist staff

The full-time Asian Link Officer and the Bereavement Officer for black and ethnic minority groups are able to communicate in local community languages and educate staff and outside agencies (for example, instructing crematorium staff that Christian crosses are not always appropriate) on specific cultural and ethnic rituals and practices, such as modesty, funeral arrangements, caring for the child's body. One of the posts is jointly funded by the local *and* health authorities. These officers raise, on a day-to-day basis, issues of concern and make suggestions for improving the delivery of the hospice service so as to reduce the numbers of mistakes staff can make in looking after families from minority ethnic communities.

Staff selection

It is seen as essential – *not* an optional extra – to have staff from various faiths and cultures. It is acknowledged that it is not easy to secure applications from suitably experienced staff, although the Equal Opportunities Policy welcomes staff from all backgrounds to apply.

Selection interviews explore attitudes in prospective employees towards people from minority ethnic communities. All application forms are 'equal opportunities' in style.

The nursing bank encourages staff from different cultural backgrounds to work at Acorns. Permanent posts have, on occasion, been filled from these staff. The 14 members of the community team range in ethnicity and can work with specific families, if necessary.

Volunteer staff recruitment

A poster campaign in different Asian languages and with appropriate pictures, resulted in several new volunteers being recruited from minority ethnic communities.

Training

Training is seen as a vital ingredient in ensuring an ethnically-sensitive service from all levels of staff. *All* new staff – paid and volunteer – undertake a one-day equal opportunities and race awareness training course led by members of Acorns. Ideally, it is felt that this could be extended to a two-to-three-day course, as frequently new staff are being trained who have a very low level of awareness.

Serious commitment to the issues covered is improved by the courses being facilitated 'in-house' rather than importing outside trainers. A powerful message of 'all faiths and cultures are welcomed here' is projected.

Policies

A firm Equal Opportunities Policy is seen as an essential point of reference for staff. A copy of the policy is made available to all new staff. The value given to these issues is emphasised, as the Director of Care Services sees all new staff and covers three core areas: training, gender issues and commitment to equal opportunities.

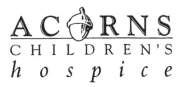

ACORNS
CHILDREN'S
h o s p i c e

Acorns looks after children with terminal illnesses and provides support for their families

Would you like to help us on a voluntary basis for a few hours a week?

আপনি কি একজন স্বেচ্ছাসেবী হিসাবে আমাদেরকে প্রতি সপ্তাহে অল্প কয়েক ঘন্টার জন্য সাহায্য করতে চান?

શું સ્વયંસેવક તરીકે અઠવાડિયામાં અમુક કલાક માટે અમને મદદ કરવાની તમારી ઇચ્છા છે?

क्या आप हर सप्ताह कुछ घंटों के लिए स्वेच्छा (वौलंटीअर) के आधार पर हमारी सहायता करना चाहेंगे?

ਕੀ ਤੁਸੀਂ ਹਰ ਹਫ਼ਤੇ ਕੁਝ ਘੰਟਿਆਂ ਲਈ ਸਵੈ-ਇੱਛਕ (ਵਲੰਟੀਅਰ) ਤੌਰ ਤੇ ਸਾਡੀ ਸਹਾਇਤਾ ਕਰਨਾ ਚਾਹੋਗੇ ?

کیا آپ رضا کارانہ بنیادوں پر ہفتے میں چند گھنٹے ہماری مدد کرنا پسند کریں گے۔

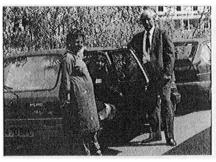

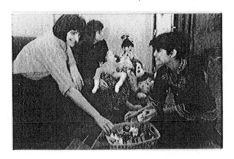

We need skilled people to run children's activities, plus drivers, gardeners, cooks, housekeepers, receptionists, maintenance people, clerical people, Asian language speakers and people willing to help our families at home.

We also run Charity shops and fund-raising activities where your help is needed.

For more information please contact:

আরো খবরাখবরের জন্য অনুগ্রহ করে যোগাযোগ করুন:

વધારે માહિતી માટે કૃપા કરી આમનો સંપર્ક સાધો:

अधिक जानकारी के लिए कृप्या इन से सम्पर्क करें

ਹੋਰ ਜਾਣਕਾਰੀ ਲਈ ਕਿਰਪਾ ਕਰਕੇ ਇਿਹਨਾਂ ਨਾਲ ਸੰਪਰਕ ਕਰੋ:

مزید معلومات کے لیے برائے مہربانی ان سے رابطہ کریں۔

TheVolunteer Co-Ordinator,
ACORNS CHILDREN'S HOSPICE,
103 Oak Tree Lane, Selly Oak, Birmingham B29 6HZ
Tel: 0121-414 1741   Fax: 0121-471 2880

Environment

Care is taken to ensure that the environment is acceptable. For example, pictures depicting certain animals which might be offensive to some faiths are avoided. The decor and pictures displayed are appealing and are those with which families from minority ethnic communities can identify. Occasionally, there are photographs along the walls of outings and celebrations at the hospice as well as groups enjoying themselves, e.g. the Asian Women's Group.

Care is taken to provide specific amenities, e.g. memorial gardens, bidets, etc. Some of these innovations were the direct result of listening to the views of the Asian women in particular, e.g. blinds over glass doors and windows in the swimming pool area to allow Asian mothers to feel more comfortable.

Crucial to the welcome and hospitality of the hospice is for visitors to see staff from a wide range of ethnicities and cultures and much emphasis is put on this aspect by senior staff.

Specific requirements

Language

It is considered essential that families are provided with skilled interpreters (Haworth et al., 1997). Staff members or outside interpreters are frequently used to avoid the use of family members to interpret. Because of the sensitive nature of the work, it is invaluable having the input from the link officers for interpretation for particularly difficult situations, although their main role is not to act as interpreters.

Much of the cost of interpreters is covered by arrangement with the local authority but substantial costs are met by the hospice itself to ensure a good-quality interpretation service is available.

Written material is not automatically translated. A message appears on the reverse of the hospice documents saying that an Interpreting Service is available.

Diets

Food is prepared appropriately according to the specific dietary requirement. In addition, there are freezer supplies so that parents can help themselves as necessary.

Modesty

Great care is taken over modesty (see 'Environment'). The hospice has been very receptive to comments and feedback from the consumers of its services, for example, over the positioning of security cameras and privacy in the pool area.

Religion

Acorns does not have a 'resident' number of religious leaders but the policy and practice is that staff work with local contacts as necessary. Detailed requirements such as the bed facing Mecca, for example, must be sensitively negotiated with those concerned. The extensive community development work in the early stages of the hospice, bore fruit in terms of the numerous contacts established.

Music, videos and books

A range of cassettes, books and videos are available in a variety of Asian languages. The availability of television channels, including Asian stations, is appreciated by the communities.

Recording and care plans

A package is used for care planning. Details of the ethnicity and language of the child and of the parent are recorded separately and whether they are spoken and/or written. This information is recorded for all main carers, the child and siblings.

Care is also taken in respecting forms of address. A note is made regarding how a letter should be addressed and to whom.

Flexibility of care

Respecting the patterns of other communities is essential to adapt the service around their needs. For example, respite care arrangements need to be flexible (i.e. frequently of six weeks' duration) as many Asian families return to their homeland for a six-week period. Care can be given to the ill child as well as to his or her siblings at the hospice, therefore respecting family bonds. For example, volunteers would be prepared to work with brothers and sisters together in the same family group.

There is no automatic allocation of 'same ethnicity' staff to patient. The flexibility of who nurses who is vital in that not all Asian people would wish to have an Asian nurse.

Groupwork

An Asian Mother's Group is well established and meets regularly. Groupwork consists of hospice-based discussion or outings. Trust and confidence in the hospice has been consolidated as a result of the group. As mentioned earlier, the views expressed by the group have been significant in shaping the service.

In order to gain the trust of the fathers, the male community worker has more recently begun to facilitate a group of fathers. It is important to be sensitive to the relationship between the influence of the paternal grandmother and mother of the child.

Future developments

As the service continues to develop, it is desirable to extend the race awareness training, to undertake community development to help other communities (e.g. Chinese) use the hospice, and to increase the Link Officer posts by two to include a male Asian officer.

A centre for people facing the challenge of AIDS

Barbara Disney, Assessment and Care Co-ordinator, London Lighthouse

A community service

London Lighthouse was the first residential and support centre for men and women affected by HIV and AIDS. Opened in 1988, London Lighthouse comprises a three-storey building in west London which was designed and commissioned solely for the purpose of providing care and support services for people infected and affected by HIV and AIDS.

The centre provides a residential facility of 21 beds, day care, a Support and Information Service, a volunteer home support service and a training facility. The ground floor has open access whilst the first floor's day centre and offices, and the second floor's residential unit have restricted access.

The entire ground floor of London Lighthouse is open to the public and the local community. It comprises a cafe, a drop-in facility and the Support and Information Service. This is open to people with HIV, family, friends and others and the various sitting areas ensure a comfortable environment. The crèche facilitates attendance at meetings and groups. A beautiful garden is, in part, geared to those with visual impairment.

There are a number of classes of different sorts to which the public have access. Good use is made of the facilities which immediately opens them up to the public. It is interesting to remember that the original vision of Dame Cicely Saunders, the pioneer of hospice and palliative care, was that units should be open to the world. However, London Lighthouse is not seen so much as a palliative care unit – although palliative care is in part what is on offer – but as a resource for services for anyone with HIV and those affected by HIV, that is, partners, families and friends. This would appear to diminish the identity as a place just for the dying, through open access, which demystifies what goes on within the walls and strengthens the relationship between London Lighthouse and the gay community particularly.

In terms of the physical nature of the building, London Lighthouse is an example of modern, friendly architecture. The plethora of notices on notice boards in the ground floor announcing community activities and providing health information emphasise the market-place atmosphere of the public area. The residential unit offers single and shared rooms. One overnight room and a flat are available for visitors. A double room is available where partners are both HIV positive. A safe environment is created for women in the residential unit and day care facility. Several small rooms permit privacy for residents and their visitors.

Residential service users are primarily white, gay men but the numbers of women (in 1996, 12.4 per cent), heterosexual men, those from minority ethnic groups (in 1996, 11.1 per cent) and those with drug and alcohol dependency are increasing in number. However, across all services at London Lighthouse, residential and non-residential, these figures are higher, with women comprising over 30 per cent of all service users.

Good practice at London Lighthouse

This service is chosen as an example of good practice with an oppressed, minority group of people living with HIV and AIDS and as it has evolved a particularly 'user friendly', accessible and appropriate service. In addition, it serves a client group other than people with cancer, who have, hitherto, been the majority of palliative care recipients. In terms of the purchaser-provider split, London Lighthouse is providing services that are positioned between care services in the community and acute medical services.

As in all good palliative care, London Lighthouse recognises that any services provided should be person-centred, the individual becomes the centre of decision making around the disease process and their concerns and worries become top priority.

The structure for developing accessible and appropriate services are clear within London Lighthouse's vision statement. It contains two main aims:

1. To provide high-quality care and support, in centres and in people's homes, empowering those with HIV and AIDS to live and die well
2. To promote the changing attitude to HIV and AIDS and to ensure the development of good public policy and service provision for affected people.

These aims are supported by four commitments:

1. To make sure that people living with HIV and AIDS are central to the organisation, so they can influence policies, develop services and actively contribute to the decision-making process
2. To create safe and welcoming environments which offer time and space to meet the needs of service users, carers and unpaid staff and visitors
3. To challenge the denial of death – to bring the issue of death into the open and recognise that it is part of life and living
4. To challenge oppression, discrimination and prejudice, promote equal opportunities and to speak up for social justice.

The vision statement and its aims are the main point of reference to any aspect of policy making and care provided at London Lighthouse.

This section focuses on how the Assessment and Care Team at London Lighthouse has been developed to promote accessible and appropriate services for this specific population.

Assessment and care team

This team of three workers acts as a bridge and gateway in reaching out to newly referred people. Following assessment, the team negotiates admission to the residential unit. Respite care is provided in episodes of one or two weeks, as supported by the individual's care manager. Convalescence/rehabilitation care is provided in two-week episodes. Terminal care is also provided.

The whole process carefully respects service users' individuality, maximises accessibility and increases the appropriateness of the care given by the unit as a result of a thorough investigation of circumstances and information gathering on needs and wishes and assessment. The team works on the basis that everything that happens with an individual, happens with their consent and involvement.

Confidentiality

London Lighthouse adheres to a strict practice of confidentiality in order to preserve good basic professional practices and in view of the sensitive nature of residents' conditions. Measures are taken to ensure that anyone in

Guidelines for using the centre

So that we can provide a safe, welcoming and comfortable environment - as free from stress as possible - there are some rules about using the centre. These apply to everyone involved with Lighthouse, including paid and unpaid staff, visitors and people who use any of our services.

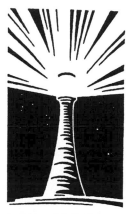

London **Lighthouse**

You may be asked to leave London Lighthouse if you do the following here.

- If you physically or verbally abuse someone. (People have the right not to experience discrimination, threats or violence, racial or sexual harassment, abuse about their sexuality, or abuse about their ability or disability.)

- If you steal or deliberately damage anything.

- If you use, deal or share street drugs (drugs which are not prescribed for you and which you cannot buy at a pharmacy).

- If you pester people for money or cigarettes.

- If you drink alcohol without getting permission first. (Permission is usually only given when alcohol is available for special occasions.)

- If you smoke in non-smoking areas.

- If you tell someone about confidential information you saw, heard or read here.

If you break any of these rules, you may be banned from the centre for a certain period or forever, or from using part or all of the centre. You may of course appeal against any decision which you feel is unfair.

the residential unit feels safe. The resident has total control over who he or she sees. Anyone wishing to visit enquires at Reception who, in turn, contacts the unit to check if the visitor is acceptable. If a visit is declined the visitor is merely told the person 'is not available' and no confirmation is given as to whether the person is a resident or not.

A similar procedure is adopted with telephone calls. When staff receive new referrals of people, care is taken in obtaining telephone numbers to check if it is safe to leave a message at the specific number given.

During the assessment process, individuals sign to give authority for information about them to be disclosed.

Referrals and assessment

Assessments of new referrals can be made within 24 hours by a member of the Assessment and Care Team, dependent on the needs and wishes of the individual referred. Each person referred has their HIV status confirmed. Careful clarifications are made with individuals referred, for example, 'How would you like to be known?', a question which respects confidentiality as well as individuality. Substantial information is amassed prior to a person entering the residential unit to have needs identified and for staff to be fully prepared for a new resident.

The front page of the referral form includes other specific information such as first language and if translation or interpretation is required. It indicates sensitivity to those whose first language is not English. Ethnic monitoring details are taken. Later in the assessment process, religious and spiritual beliefs, ethnicity and dietary needs are identified and recorded. In the current climate where funding has been disaggregated from the one 'host purchasing' authority to the seven Inner London Health Authorities, each with separate contracts, the assessment process has become increasingly stringent in ascertaining relevant pre-admission information.

This involves increased liaison with medical teams, local authority social services care managers and other agencies and runs the risk of the perception of a person's needs being coloured by others' views. This can be seen as undermining the individual's view of themselves and their needs. To counterbalance this danger, staff are quick to ensure that when new residents arrive, they are given an opportunity to express their views.

New documentation has been developed to encompass the many aspects of a person and their care needs. This allows the individual being assessed to identify and actively contribute. Their signature confirms the statement of needs.

Once the person enters the residential unit, the Assessment and Care Team conducts a mid-way review of their needs and plans for discharge, liaising closely with the care managers concerned.

Contracts

If it is assessed that a resident is likely to pose problems, he or she is asked to sign a 'contract' acknowledging that residents have responsibilities requiring limits on certain behaviours and displays of attitudes relating to drugs, alcohol or racism. This endeavours to place boundaries on behaviour to ensure a safe environment for other residents and for staff.

Staff

Staff do not wear uniform but name badges, in an attempt to break down barriers between staff and residents. Staff members – men and women – range across ethnicity, sexual orientation and religious affiliation, endeavouring to give a clear message of openness and diversity.

When a new resident arrives, a nurse meets them at Reception and gives them a personal welcome. Each resident is cared for by a particular team of nurses. Nurses are not allocated on a 'matched' basis, e.g. black nurse to black resident, etc., except for women residents where a request for same gender is respected.

Volunteers

With more than 350 volunteers working with London Lighthouse, there are opportunities for involvement from the local and wider community, breaking down barriers between a specialist service and the lay public. As with other services, volunteers not only provide skilled help but become ambassadors for the service, supporting fund-raising events and other related activities. The Home Support Service is staffed mainly by volunteers (200) visiting individuals at home.

The Volunteer Co-ordinator prioritises service users for volunteer posts (e.g. reception) and, of the 160 volunteers currently working in the building, 24 per cent are HIV positive. This is just one example of service user ownership.

User participation

The founders' conviction was that people with HIV and AIDS should have control over their lives and contribute in making key decisions about the organisation, its quality and its range of services. It is this user involvement and partnership approach that makes London Lighthouse so 'user friendly'.

The philosophy that 'everything that happens to someone happens with their consent' is well respected. Nurses spend considerable time with residents talking through what is happening to them medically and emotionally and to listening to their views. London Lighthouse's welcome brochure states, 'Share your views ... have your say. We respond to the needs of people using the service and aim to ensure that your voices are heard both inside our organisation and in the wider world.'

A system of mid-stay interviews are being introduced whereby a member of the Assessment and Care Team will meet with the resident to ensure that their needs jointly identified at assessment are being met.

A Service Users' Consultative forum meets every six weeks. This affords the opportunity for *any* service user to meet members of the Senior Management Team and the Chief Executive, thus ensuring service users' views are heard. Additionally, there are ten Service Users' Representatives. These individuals are invited to sit on internal working groups – for example, the press strategy working group, access to the ground floor working group, and feedback to the Service Users' Consultative Forum – providing another mechanism for ensuring service users are heard and needs met. Additionally, the representatives have a rota where they are 'on duty' to offer peer support and can represent individuals who may have a complaint or particular issue they wish to address. Various changes have been made as a result of this process, e.g. removing all the mirrors in the lifts!

Service users are always on the panel for open mornings alongside departmental heads. Further, London Lighthouse's complaints procedure is clear in encouraging service users in making use of the procedure.

Open access

The centre is not only open to the public but residents have open access to counsellors, complementary therapists, dietetic advice, occupational therapists and physiotherapists. Residents are free to choose where to eat, either on the residential unit or in the cafe, again mixing with staff members and members of the local community.

A number of classes occur throughout the week where residents, staff and the public can attend without having to identify their particular role. This is levelling and empowering as it allows the residents, staff member or visitor to just be themselves and relate in their own right. Activities involve recreational pursuits, the AIDS quilt making, relaxation and entertainment.

London Lighthouse is also a venue for community groups to meet, thus attracting visitors and breaking down barriers further.

General observations

London Lighthouse has pioneered novel ways of caring for a particular group of people in a setting where palliative care principles of individuality, respect, confidentiality, family and friends as the unit of care, a person-centred approach and good symptom control act as the basis of the service. Maximum accessibility is allowed by evolving services that are appropriate to the community of people with HIV and AIDS. It is clearly a setting different from the average palliative care service which works with people generally much more ill and with a high proportion of deaths occurring in the unit. For example, user participation is likely to be somewhat easier in a population who are articulate, less likely to be in a terminal phase of illness and less stuck in the 'grateful patient' syndrome.

A multi-faith hospice

Jane Thomson, Social Work Director, North London Hospice

As hospices and palliative care units have grown in large numbers around the country and addressed the needs of their local populations, the need to alter radically the architecture and facilities, and to some extent attitude, according to the communities being served, became apparent. As the first multi-faith hospice, how has the North London Hospice achieved its task in practice?

A 20-bed independent hospice with day centre and home care service set up on multi-faith lines, the hospice serves the London boroughs of Barnet, Enfield and Haringey. This contains a population of approximately 750,000 and a very mixed area culturally, ethnically and religiously (approximately 30 per cent are minority ethnic communities). About 25 per cent of the population of Barnet, the borough in which the hospice is situated, is Jewish.

Background

In 1984 the then North London Hospice Group came together with members of the Jewish community and planned to open a hospice catering for people of all faiths and for those of no 'formal faith'. It was strongly felt that religious and spiritual needs of patients and families should be met 'as of right' and people should not be made to feel guests. The pioneers were very aware of the Christian, white, middle-class image of the hospice movement, especially in the early 1980s and considered this inappropriate for the catchment area to be served.

An accessible building

The hospice has aimed to create spaces that individuals and families can use according to their own preferences.

Rooms

Twelve out of the 20 beds are in single rooms with own shower/WC; this facilitates the privacy and respect for patients and their families living for a period in the hospice in their own style (own objects and rituals, prayers, extended family visiting, personal hygiene, relatives having more choice at how long the body is left in the room after death, etc.).

Kitchens

Kosher and Halal kitchens are available in the ward area for use by relatives and appropriate dietary requirements can be met by the main hospice kitchen.

Prayer and reading rooms

A small prayer room is furnished suitably for all faiths and includes appropriate objects and religious texts. This is used for quiet prayer or for small services. From early days it was important to model different terminology from the traditional, for example, 'prayer room' rather than 'chapel'. The stained glass commissioned is based on nature and emphasises the continuity of life. The challenge for such a project is overcoming the risk of the room being seen by some as too bland, yet appealing to the commonality of the faiths. It is difficult to create an atmosphere that is prayerful and yet welcoming to all faiths. This is still being developed.

Adjacent to the prayer room is a reading room containing a wide range of reading material of a religious and spiritual nature. The rooms look onto the 'Tree of Life' sculpture symbol especially commissioned for the hospice and emphasising its multi-faith nature.

Viewing room in mortuary

This contains an especially designed bed which is versatile and can meet the requirements of many faiths, for example, to face Mecca or to be lowered. A range of religious objects is also available to be used according to the needs of the family and religious community.

Pictures

There is no specific religious decor on the walls of the hospice and care is taken that no offensive pictures are displayed, for example, depicting certain animals.

Staff

Interviews for new staff and volunteers always raise questions about attitudes towards working with people from different cultures and consideration is given to new staff fitting into the way of working of the multi-professional team. Great care is taken to guard against employing people who wish to use the hospice as a basis for proselytising.

Occasionally second interviews have taken place to ensure that attitudes would be consistent with the ethos of the hospice.

Policy and procedures

Clearly established standards and expectations are necessary to ensure paid and volunteer staff know what is expected of them. For example, on admission procedures, staff are reminded not to make assumptions regarding preferences of patients. It is important to ensure that the work practices and procedures are supportive of the concepts inherent in the culture of the hospice.

Training

Formal and careful induction training of new staff reinforces fundamental practices. 'Training' comes from patients who share information about rituals and family traditions.

There is an interest from staff to understand the different faiths and cultures. On all major festivals and holy days, the appropriate religious leader will talk about the significance of the event. An 'oral tradition' of more experienced colleagues passing information to others is thought to be valuable. This emphasis on colleagues helping each other and passing on 'the way things are done' is seen as good practice, over and above training courses.

Multi-faith chaplaincy

Patients in the hospice are visited by any one of the chaplaincy team on duty, not necessarily of their own faith, unless specially requested. Patients not wanting to have a visit are equally respected. The team comprises members of Church of England, Free Church, Hindu, Jewish (Orthodox, Reform and Masorti), Muslim and Roman Catholic faiths; they are all unpaid. A Jewish rabbi co-ordinates the team but this role has rotated between its different members. The chaplains (there is still a no more acceptable multi-faith term) try to respond to people and their suffering on a spiritual dimension as well as supporting the patient in their own faith.

As with paid staff, the appointment of the right personality and skill base is essential. Therefore, chaplains are appointed by the management team and approved by the hospice council.

Pastoral group

A group comprising representatives of all the main faiths and humanists meets three times a year and acts as an outreach to their faith communities. This has been an excellent way of reaching out to the different communities and building credibility with churches, synagogues and other places of worship. The group meeting is also an important means of the senior staff of the hospice ensuring that the direction and ethos of the pastoral input is in keeping with the overall aims and philosophy of the hospice.

In such a sensitive area, this group has been through the usual stages of 'norming', 'storming' and 'reforming' in becoming a viable group. Initially there was concern not to offend; the group was outnumbered by Christian clergy; many in the group had never sat in the same room or 'done business' with a member of another faith, for example, Hindu or Muslim, as a colleague.

One of many turning points was an evening visit and reception at the hospice targeted at all local religious leaders and faith communities. Soon after the in-patient unit opened, the hospice was dedicated by a group of five national leaders representing the major faiths.

Creating a database of religious groups and communities was a challenge, as little information currently existed and making personal contact was crucial. Timing of meetings is also a factor to be considered, not only on account of religious requirements, but also because many lay or religious leaders of the minority faiths have paid jobs during the day.

Multi-faith seminars

Several successful seminars have been organised by the Pastoral Group in an attempt to understand how death and bereavement are perceived in the different belief systems. Examples of themes explored include 'Someone has died: what has happened?' and 'If there is a God, why did He or She let this happen?'

Working in a multi-cultural way

Integral to the hospice's philosophy is the fostering of understanding and acceptance between different community groups. This must begin with staff learning from each other.

A 'Thought for the Day' time for staff, on a weekly basis, led by either staff or chaplains, allows for some mutual understanding and team building. A planned development is a 'Thought for the Season', to involve more staff. These initiatives help to respond to the danger of the concept of 'multi-faith' becoming 'no faith'.

There is a real danger that such a strong emphasis on mutual respect may render bland and 'watered down' the experience of the different faiths. The North London Hospice has created a rich environment. A dilemma is 'bending over backwards to accommodate others', yet supporting spiritual life in becoming live and real.

Developing a multi-faith service requires constant working. For example, there still remains proportionately few black or Asian patients or staff, and education and development of staff is ongoing.

In terms of individual practice some of the professional challenges include: listening to what patients and families from other cultures really want and getting beyond politeness; working with the limitations of interpreters unused to the work; the gender of the worker involved, and continuous trust-building with different communities. Translating and interpreting the multi-faith ideal into some everyday reality for individual patients keeps the concept dynamic and not merely a professional conceptualisation.

Summary of good practice

Understanding the ill person's culture

In order to understand a person you need to understand his or her culture. However, this becomes complicated as we tend to see the world through our own culture and norms.

Our own culture will colour the way we assess the particular needs of people from other cultures (Oliviere, 1993). We must clearly never assume our own culture or a eurocentric perspective is the norm but try to appreciate the values, norms and attitudes of the other person.

When we work with any individual or group, especially when there are obvious differences, we must take into account the world views that might be affecting the cultures of the professional or patient and family.

Values

Individuality - Groupness
Independence - Interdependence
Uniqueness - Sameness
Difference - Community

Experience

Separate - Integration
Concrete - Abstract
Material - Spiritual
Control over nature - - - - - - - - - - - - - - - - - - At one with nature
Competition - Co-operation

Intervention

Individual rights - - - - - - - - - - - - - - - - - Collective responsibility
Explain - Discover
Activity - Inactivity

(Based on Stjernsward, J. (1995) lecture to British Council students, London

Fig. 7.1   World views and culture

These concepts and values on the continua above are not in themselves right or wrong states. They are largely based on eastern and western perspectives but, as we are all a mixture, it is important that we locate ourselves and our families in order to have an appreciation of them and their needs.

The above framework reinforces the need to get to know the ill person and his family rather than relying on assumption and one's own world view. We must be aware, too, that some people from other cultures may be uncomfortable with a more westernised medical approach to consulting patients. Also, knowledge of a particular culture can be a dangerous thing as we can presume certain information rather than use it to know which questions to ask.

A number of recent publications are useful in promoting ethnically and culturally sensitive practice (Green, 1991, 1993; Lothian Racial Equality Council, 1992, Gunaratnam, 1993; Neuberger, 1994; O'Neill, 1994; Cancerlink, 1995b; Salamagne and Keunebroek, 1996).

Despite all the principles listed, good practice in achieving accessible and appropriate palliative care services will only be experienced if the stated policies and practices are in harmony, the patients and families are made to feel welcomed and their views are listened to and acted upon. At a basic level, these practices are no different to meeting the needs of any group but with certain communities, the fundamentals of good practice become essential.

Table 7.1 **Framework for achieving accessible and appropriate palliative care services**

	Principle	*Practice*
Mission statement	Commitment to equality in value base and in stated aims.	All staff aware.
Policy and procedures	Management committed. Equal Opportunities Policy.	Staff clear on expectations. Staff and Service users understand.
Staff selection	Staff matching ethos. Community participation as volunteers.	Careful selection. Diversity of staff – paid and unpaid.
Training	Skilled workforce.	Induction and ongoing training. Annual appraisal.
Environment	User-friendly/ hospitable/trust.	Furnishings and decor reducing unfamiliarity.
Written material	Good communication.	Understandable language/ offer of interpreter.
Language	Good communication.	Prepare list of interpreters. Training/debriefing essential. Consider health advocates.
Community development	Trust building. Equal access.	Personal contact. Identify community leaders. Visits to unit. Work with local GPs. Use community's own media.
Ethnic monitoring	Information on those currently accessing.	Incorporating into database. Staff training vital.
Patient notes	Accurate information to plan care.	Record first language spoken/written name, dietary, religious requirements, family.
Resources	Patient comfort.	Availability of books, cassettes with appropriate images and language.
Diet	Good care.	Availability of other foods.
Pastoral care	Respect for individuals.	Develop contacts from main faiths. Ensure training.
Personal care	Individuality and respect.	Staff understanding of gender, modesty, personal hygiene.

Table 7.1   *continued*

Family and community	Support for patient's network.	Understand culture of wider family, death and bereavement customs and rituals.
Bereavement	Prevention.	Discerning culturally appropriate patterns from risk. Counsellors from local communities.
Feedback and evaluation	Service improvement	Seeking views. Consulting individuals and groups. User and carer participation.

Achieving accessible and appropriate services

This chapter has considered the way palliative care services are planned, structured and delivered to ensure they are as accessible and appropriate as possible for people whose culture, for whatever reason, has marked differences from the majority. In practical terms, this is often particularly important to people from minority ethnic communities because of problems of language and discrimination, but the same good practice principles apply to people from other groups in the community.

Culture should not be viewed as a singular concept, but rather as incorporating 'institutions, language, values, religious ideals, habits of thinking, artistic expressions, and patterns of social and interpersonal relationships' (Lum, 1992).

The concept of cultural pain is infrequently talked about in palliative care and it may be more subtle than other dimensions in the total pain framework, but it is nevertheless real. A palliative care service or practitioner who neglects cultural issues, could be disenfranchising many from accessing the care they need.

Resources

African-Caribbean Mental Health Association (ACMHA) 35–37 Electric Avenue, Brixton, London SW9 8JP Tel: 0171 737 3603. Therapeutic and legal issues, volunteer befriending and advocacy

AIDS Helpline Tel: 0800 567123

Asian Family Counselling Service 74 The Avenue, Ealing, London W13 8LB Tel: 0181 997 5749. Marital and family counselling for the Asian community

Black HIV/AIDS Forum Zion Community Resource Centre, Zion Crescent, Hulme, Manchester, M15 5BY

Blackliners Unit 46, Eurolink Centre, 49 Effra Road, London SW2 1BZ Tel: 0171 738 7468 (Admin) 0171 738 5274 (Helpline).
A voluntary organisation run by black people for black people of African, Asian and Caribbean descent, affected by AIDS. Support services include domiciliary care and befriending

Cancer Black Care 18 Ashwin Street, London E8 3DL. Tel: 0171 249 1097
Addresses cultural and emotional care of black people affected by cancer and includes their carers, family and friends

Health Education Authority 'Caring for Patients' Published by Health Education Authority in association with Help the Hospices. A fully illustrated multilingual guide to common medical problems and procedures

Nafsiyat Inter-cultural Therapy Centre 278 Seven Sisters Road, Finsbury Park, London N1 2HY Tel: 0171 263 4130. Psychotherapy and counselling to black people and people from ethnic minorities

SHAP Calendar of Religious Festivals SHAP Working Party, c/o The National Society's R.E. Centre, 36 Causton Street, London SW1P 4AU Tel: 0171 932 1194

8 Working with volunteers

'I thought that I was going to be the icing on the cake, but there are days when I feel more like the contents of the mixing bowl.'
(A hospice volunteer)

Volunteers give their time and energy to perform acts of public service without financial remuneration and it is estimated that there are about six million deployed in the United Kingdom at the present time. The promotion and development of volunteering was an important strategy in the Major government's plans for implementing community care; however, although there are strong traditions of using volunteers in hospices, NHS hospitals used proportionately fewer volunteers with more restricted roles. With a few notable exceptions, social services departments, whose care managers have responsibility for assessing and contracting social services for people with life-threatening illness, have been either less enthusiastic or less successful in recruiting them. In a report on volunteering produced by the Department of Health's Social Services Inspectorate (1996), four out of six social services departments were found to be 'concerned chiefly with purchasing and contracting with voluntary bodies than with the promotion of volunteering'. The sample was very small but the report did draw attention to the potential difficulties of integrating the deployment of volunteers into the work of care managers. It is worth noting therefore that this is not an area of palliative care which deploys volunteers to any great extent at present.

The examples from which it is intended to identify issues and extract principles of good practice are the Child Death Helpline and the work of a voluntary services co-ordinator (VSC) at a mainstream hospice. (See also Chapter 6 'Bereavement care' and Relf and Couldrick, 1988.)

The Child Death Helpline

Jean Simons, Bereavement Services Co-ordinator, Great Ormond Street NHS Trust Hospital for Sick Children, London.

This service is offered through the co-operative efforts of the two children's hospitals, the Great Ormond Street Hospital in London and the Alder Centre at the Alder Hey Children's Hospital in Liverpool, the latter having pioneered a helpline and drop-in centre as a service for people affected by the death of a child, mainly in the North of England, some eight years ago. About five years ago, Great Ormond Street (GOS) decided to offer a similar service in the South of England. It soon became clear from the response that a national, co-ordinated service was needed. The information below describes the arrangements at the London (GOS) base, but the philosophy of the service and approach to training applies to both centres.

The Child Death Helpline (CDH) is located within the Great Ormond Street Hospital's bereavement services department, which offers assessment and counselling to bereaved families, contributes to policy development and implementation in the hospital, undertakes training of all grades of professional staff and volunteers and provides supervision for staff and volunteers. The Child Death Helpline comprises the joint co-ordinators, an administrator, approximately 40 bereaved parent volunteers and professionals and a small group of professional supervisors. The helpline, by using the services of volunteers based at the centres, is able to operate on a nationwide basis, via a freephone number. This in itself is an achievement but what makes this project an interesting example of practice is the way in which it has given real power to bereaved parents by involving them in equal numbers to professionals from the planning stages and by recruiting them to run the telephone helpline with professional support and supervision. The project is also located in a department which presses for parental choice in matters relating to the death of a child and in areas where hospitals often have their own unchallenged procedures and practices: for example, the parents may wish to take the child's body home (in preference to having it placed in the hospital mortuary), which is perfectly legal so long as the death certificate has been signed and a corner's post-mortem is not required. The bereavement services department also makes great efforts, through educating and training staff including the telephone volunteers, to ensure that parents are really well-informed about giving consent to post-mortem and in the matter of organ donation. Care is also taken to ensure that staff are aware of the special arrangements which need to be taken in order to meet the religious requirements of the main faiths.

The philosophy of the department is first to work in a genuine partnership with parents and second to be pro-active in seeking to make parental choice a reality in all matters to do with child death. The Child Death Helpline has a joint management committee representing the two locations, though it has just the one freephone telephone number. The helpline is open seven evenings and three mornings per week, staffed by volunteers from both centres.

The service was established because help for bereaved parents was 'patchy' across the country, with hospital practices varying enormously; parents might be distressed about what they had been told was or was not possible, but tended to accept 'rules' as stated. The emphasis on parental choice came directly out of feedback from parents about their experiences and it became clear that a new culture was needed within hospitals which were caring for children with life-threatening illness, extending into the period after death.

No deliberate obstacles were placed before the group who were committed to establishing this new approach (at Great Ormond Street Hospital, this was the Terminal Care Group), but rather an inability to understand why such high levels of consultation and acquiescence with parents' wishes were considered to be essential to good practice. There tended to be a 'paternalistic' view that parents may 'not cope' with the kind of choices and decisions the group wanted to introduce. Amongst all professionals there were one or two who displayed a willingness to decide what parents' needs were, without much exploration of them and some (notably among doctors) who would typically say 'They seem to be managing very well to me ... I always tell them that they can ring me.'

It was therefore an 'innocence' of existing emotional need rather than active opposition which had to be overcome. Eventually, it was the increasingly positive feedback from parents who had been helped by a more open attitude, that gradually brought about the new culture, initially reinforced by knowledge of established good practice in relation to still-birth and maternity units.

It is unlikely that these changes could have come about if the initiators had not established their own professional credibility over many years and been willing to commit a good deal of time to working with the relevant groups in the hospital in order to engage the interest of key people, promote changes and support arguments with the relevant research. The changes must also have been aided however, by an established tradition of innovation in the hospital (in this case Great Ormond Street Hospital) which pioneered a Symptom Care Team (for those caring for a child dying at home) and appointed the country's first Paediatric Palliative Care Consultant.

Key steps in realising the practice

As the 'new culture' had begun to be established, it was possible to gain support for the idea of a helpline planned and run by parents to be located within a co-ordinated bereavement services department. It was then necessary for the initiating professionals and bereaved parents to become involved personally in committees and working groups so that the concept of working in partnership could become an accepted way of working. Part of the process was an increasing contribution from many members of these groups on how they might extend the areas of parental participation and decision making. The role of the professional (who ultimately became the co-ordinator of the bereavement services department in this case) was to encourage implementation and monitoring. Alongside this process the regular reference to research and literature which supported the proposed changes continued.

A steering committee (later the bereavement working group of the CDH) was set up to establish the helpline and thus the crucial principle of having equal numbers of parents and professionals in partnership was implemented from the outset.

Basic principles involved in establishing this kind of practice

The primary principle is that of equal responsibility between parents and professionals in decision making and a related principle is that of abandoning professional paternalism in favour of a pro-active determination to empower parents. The amalgamation of the service at the Alder Centre and the CDH at Great Ormond Street created a nationwide service: all volunteer workers had themselves experienced the death of their child and the professional role enabled these volunteers to offer the kind of service which parents had made clear they wanted.

Resource implications for setting up and maintaining the helpline

As this service is offered by means of a freephone telephone number, the expense falls on the CDH itself. In 1997 the helpline was open for 30 hours per week and the annual telephone bill was approximately £15,000. Since the service is located within two NHS Hospital Trusts, it benefits 'in kind' from office accommodation, heating, lighting, cleaning costs and so on, which are already incurred.

An independent hospice volunteer service

Joan Towle, formerly the Volunteer Services Co-ordinator, Mount Edgcumbe Hospice, St Austell, Cornwall

This example comes from Mount Edgcumbe Hospice in St Austell, Cornwall, a 21-bed hospice which offers in-patient care and day care, and is expanding its areas of home care. The authors identify the 'good practice' here as representing a thoughtful, methodical approach to the selection, training and support of volunteers in a hospice setting and one which, though untypical in several respects, provides a valuable working model.

The hospice is currently one of two serving the county and its catchment area is widespread and rural. The area attracts people in retirement as well as an annual influx of tourists. Average earnings are low compared with many other parts of the country and unemployment is also well above the national average. The population of the county is 99 per cent white.

Great care in recruitment was thought necessary for a number of reasons. The hospice movement attracts volunteers with little difficulty but amongst the applicants are those who could be unsuited and/or harmful to its work; the flexibility of hospice care and its demanding nature require particular attention to the induction and training of volunteers. In addition, the hospice movement ethos with its emphasis on understanding and acceptance of the ill person can leave volunteers in a vulnerable position unless they are provided with clear expectations, guidelines and a supportive framework of professional practice. With these prerequisites in place, it is believed that volunteers can reinforce the ill person's sense of self-worth and relieve pressure on paid staff, both of which contributions can have an enriching quality in the lives of the volunteers themselves.

There were some obstacles to be overcome initially, in terms of recruitment: for example, a public perception of hospices as 'gloomy' places which were unlikely to provide a source of rewarding or enjoyable voluntary effort. There was also ambivalence among staff, some of whom wondered if volunteers would not be 'more trouble than they were worth' and some who saw the unpaid labour as a potential solution to any problem which required 'another pair of hands'. A more difficult obstacle to overcome was establishing in principle the volunteer's need for accurate feedback on their performance, up to and including disciplinary procedures. This duty was divided between the voluntary services co-ordinator (VSC), departmental heads and those in day-to-day positions of responsibility. The most recent principle to be established was the need to maintain effective support for both the newest and longest-serving volunteer, the ages of whom ranged from 16 to 75.

The key steps in realising the practice were firstly a clear recognition of the VSC's role: this was achieved by means of a carefully thought-out job description, clarification at departmental meetings and through a range of personal contacts. It was then decided to build up the volunteer group starting with one line-manager and monitoring the deployment of the volunteer through regular contact. Another step was ensuring that the occasional early 'crisis' was identified as a source of learning for both volunteer and staff and not left as an unspoken concern. The development of written material and documentation was seen as essential to sustaining a smooth-running volunteer service, avoiding the kind of oral culture which can lead to misunderstandings. The final step was establishing and frequently reiterating the principle that the hospice has a staff group comprising paid and unpaid people – not a staff group plus volunteers. This last step meant that the staff-room where people took their breaks was for everyone and it also made it easier for volunteers to accept that the adherence to matters of confidentiality and health and safety regulations as well as the application of disciplinary measures should properly apply to them as members of the staff group.

The basic principles involved in the development of this practice have been implied to some extent in describing the key steps but they may be summarised as follows: 'That volunteers, as other staff, have both rights and responsibilities; that their role is to supplement rather than to replace paid staff; that the volunteer force will live up to what is expected of it'.

The resource implications are probably about the same as for any similar-sized hospice and include the cost of paid staff time in introducing and maintaining the volunteer workforce, that is, the cost of training and support, uniforms, insurance, an extension of staff facilities such as a changing-room to include the volunteers, an office for the VSC and of course the VSC salary, if she or he is not also a volunteer. By agreement, a variety of volunteers' expenses are also met.

Key issues

The distinction between paid and unpaid work is fairly clear. The distinction between professional and non-professional merits some exploration, however. On a continuum of skill, volunteers can be placed anywhere from changing the water in flower vases to responding personally to people who have suffered the death of their child and at the latter end, the boundaries between what is a 'professional' activity and what is 'befriending' require some clarification. The CDH highlights the issue in that the telephone work undertaken by these volunteers would undoubtedly be regarded by many professionals outside of palliative care as 'too difficult for amateurs'. The response would be that the 'professional' objective should be to ensure that those wanting help receive the kind of help they say they need and in the case of parents who have lost a child, most want to talk over their experience with others who have shared this experience. There seemed to be a perceived difference for parents between those people who could help during illness and treatment and those who could best help after the child had died. Despite child death being seen by professionals as carrying a high risk of complicated grief reaction, it is interesting to note that only a small number of callers actually went on to receive professional counselling. The professional role here is identified as a responsibility to provide what the service user wants, offering a parallel with the principle of care management. Nor is there any evidence to suggest that a person who has been bereaved *must* need or want professional counselling, even when they have lost a child. If a caller does want more than the telephone volunteer feels able to provide, then informing them about the nature and availability of professional help would be an appropriate part of the role. Recruitment and preparation for this kind of helping, as opposed to professional training, will be addressed later.

The whole of the distinction between 'professional' and 'amateur', or paid and voluntary, can become blurred in the field of palliative care. The VSC who established the volunteer force at the Mount Edgcumbe Hospice took the view that 'the staff' consisted of both paid and voluntary workers; the volunteers therefore had both rights and responsibilities in line with paid staff but appropriately framed for their differing level of involvement. For example, this means that volunteers know that they can be subject to disciplinary measures; rather than being a disincentive, many view this with approval as it means that their role is being taken seriously.

It has to be said, however, that the development of policies which may seem subtly to undermine professional security, at a time when prevailing ideologies have placed professionals under many sorts of attack, is a sensitive area. Care must be taken in blurring or overstepping of professional boundaries. It is also worth noting on this topic that some of the CDH volunteers are health or social work professionals when they are not befriending other parents, underlining the fact that 'volunteer' does not necessarily mean 'amateur' but rather 'not acting in one's professional capacity'. There are other examples of this – for instance, many Conciliation Service volunteers have a 'day job' as lawyers, social workers or probation officers.

Recruitment and selection

The recruitment and selection of volunteers in palliative care is regarded by the initiators of both the above examples as a matter requiring considerable care. Many hospice applicants are the result of 'word of mouth' in that they know or have met someone who is already a hospice volunteer. This has the advantage of informing the potential recruit about the nature of the work, the training and support, and possibly of providing some understanding of the hospice philosophy. A disadvantage, however, is that 'like tends to attract like' and too much reliance on personal contact for recruitment may result in a homogeneous group which neither reflects the resident group nor provides the mix of age, gender, culture and approach to match the tasks for which the volunteers are needed; nor, of course does it offer equal opportunity within the local community to people who may wish to volunteer their services. In the case of the CDH, the principle of believing what people say about the kind of help they need and endeavouring to provide it, does result in 'like attracting like' but only in this one crucial experience of sharing the death of a child; in every other respect the helpline volunteers are as heterogeneous as the caller group.

The hospice VSC begins recruitment with a person specification in mind and a possible deployment, though the former always outweighs the latter: that is to say that if an applicant seems to be 'right' for the hospice setting, then the co-ordinator will seek to find a place for that person to utilise their skills and meet their interests even if this means not immediately filling a particular 'gap' in the volunteer workforce. Conversely, an applicant may be very keen to work on the wards or in the day care centre which will give them maximum contact with the ill people; but if the co-ordinator feels that these roles might be too physically or emotionally demanding, or that the applicant's approach might be too forceful for these situations, an alternative role would be offered. Sometimes the distance an applicant would have to travel, or their particular skills, might make them more suitable for other activities outside the hospice itself. If nothing can be found to match their abilities, they will be referred to another voluntary organisation or the local volunteer bureau.

The question of suitability for any voluntary work is a matter of fine judgement which can, of course, be in error, but the VSC in palliative care has a responsibility to the ethos of hospice care, to the vulnerability of seriously ill people and their families and to the welfare of those who volunteer. These responsibilities do not always fit easily together. Also, although hospices have moved on from being places for the dying to being places for pain and symptom control and for helping to improve the quality of life for patients, public image lags behind. It is encouraging that they still receive such numbers of volunteer applicants, but hospices can also attract people whose motivation is complex, or occasionally questionable. It is also possible that strong religious beliefs can attract applicants to hospice work in search of converts, or the opportunity to minister to those who have not chosen such attentions and would not welcome them.

Even more careful judgement is required when motivation is beyond question, but the applicants are vulnerable. They may be looking for the warmth and caring ethos of the hospice to fill an emptiness in their own lives or seek to transfer to the hospice staff and patients the care and affection no longer needed by their own families. Such people can make the best of volunteers, but unless there is some balance between the satisfaction they gain from their volunteer role and that from the rest of their life, they can become over-dependent on and over-engaged in the work. Others can find that close involvement with death and dying people becomes more than they can cope with. The VSC must try to avoid recruiting over-vulnerable volunteers and to prevent any volunteer from becoming a responsibility to, rather than a resource for, other staff members. The volunteers should gain and be enriched, rather than suffer, as a result of their work.

Policies

Clear policies are needed in two areas where the needs of the volunteer and of the hospice may not coincide. A bereavement may leave someone with time to spare and care to give but at risk of not giving themselves time to grieve, if their caring role is transferred too quickly to volunteer caring. There has therefore grown up a tradition in many hospices not to accept applicants within two years of a major bereavement and an acknowledgement that current volunteers may need either support or a sabbatical period. Such policies clearly need to be adaptable, since in some communities, for example, gay or refugee, the experience of multiple loss may be the norm. The onset of old age for a current volunteer also leads to difficult decisions: retired people are the most available of volunteers and hospices provide safe, easily accessible working conditions – nor does chronological age equate with suitability or unsuitability. However, at some point, physical ageing and its restrictions will outweigh these factors and the VSC will have to implement a decision that will be a form of bereavement for the volunteer.

In the most general terms, the VSC, recruiting and selecting in the field of palliative care, is looking for people who are adaptable, not too committed to their own way of doing things, content to work to the instructions of others and willing to accept direction and discipline. They must be able to keep their personal views and beliefs to themselves and to relate easily to a wide range of people, often very different from themselves, with sympathy and warmth.

Role of volunteers

So far as the general role of volunteers is concerned, Joan Towle originally took the view that if any job was more than part-time, and needed continuity, it was not appropriate for a volunteer: if the kitchen needed an additional paid staff member, then that is what should be sought. This issue of replacing paid staff is highlighted by the obvious benefits of asking retired nurses, carpenters, electricians and kitchen staff to continue their work for hospices on a voluntary basis, say after retirement. This does risk however trade union opposition for depriving unemployed people of a job and it could raise serious problems about insurance or professional liability. Thus at Mount Edgcumbe Hospice an electrician will be valued as a volunteer driver but he will not be asked to repair the toaster – however convenient that would be. Against this, the willingness of people to offer not only financial support but contributions in kind, including their personal skills, lead to a large grey area where great care must be taken. Hospices are also aware that the regular volunteer component, be it only one day a week for each volunteer, to services such as day care is essential for quality of service and perhaps their financial viability. With the CDH the question of volunteers replacing paid staff does not apply in that the callers want to talk to someone who has shared their experience and this is not a form of employment. Some volunteers for the CDH may be health and social work professionals 'during the day' and whilst this may have given them a particular appreciation of the need for such a service, they may face a particular difficulty during volunteer training in learning to respond to callers simply as parents who have shared an experience rather than as professionals.

Once the volunteer has been accepted at Mount Edgcumbe Hospice for a particular role, it is the hospice policy to attach them for an initial period to a 'tutor', an experienced volunteer who can 'show them the ropes' and model an approach to the work which is appropriate. So far as is realistic, the newcomer will be given 'easy' tasks to begin with but as soon as the new recruit feels comfortable in the role and their 'tutor' and line-manager concur, they will be given their own responsibilities and treated as a member of a staff team. Nevertheless, volunteers do not have (because they do not need it) the same access to information about the patients as nursing staff; volunteers are only told what they need to know in order to carry out their tasks. The majority of residents have cancer but an increasing proportion have neurological conditions, including motor neurone disease and there are occasionally people with AIDS. It is emphasised that adherence to safe practices in working with seriously ill people is not just to protect staff but to protect the residents from potential infection from anyone who may unknowingly have hepatitis or be HIV positive. Newcomers to hospice work also need to understand that a minor infectious or contagious disorder in an otherwise healthy person can be life-threatening to someone who already has a serious condition.

Training and support

As has become evident, volunteers in palliative care not only need to be adaptable, reliable and accepting but they also need training and support. The primary objective of training is to enable the volunteer to carry out the tasks assigned to them in an effective and appropriate way and, to this extent, much of that 'teaching' will be done by the team to which they are attached, in particular by the volunteer's line-manager. There are matters which need to be understood by all volunteers, however, regardless of their specific deployment and the same training can also benefit groups such as councils or boards of management who take policy decisions. The first of these is to acquire an accurate understanding of the hospice ethos and the professional roles of its paid staff. This enables volunteers to see how they 'fit into' the overall picture and how they can supplement the services. In addition, they need to understand health and safety regulations and fire precautions which, if taught imaginatively, can make an impression and potentially save lives. It has also been found that volunteers welcome training sessions which inform them generally about the medical conditions which the hospice residents are having to deal with and what is involved in the various treatments; this will not only help the volunteer to get some idea of what the ill person may be feeling or going through but it is also an aspect of training which can be valuable in dispelling many public misconceptions about some of the illnesses encountered in hospices.

The particular part of training which is appreciated because it meets one of the primary concerns of volunteers, however, is that which focuses on conversations with the ill person. 'I shan't know what to say' is the most commonly expressed worry. Training designed to respond to this must always offer time for the volunteers to think through their concerns and consider possible ways of responding. The idea of being 'other-centred' in one's communications is not easy to grasp, even for professionals like social workers and counsellors, requiring as it does that we put our own train of thought 'on hold' and only show interest in the other's thoughts; but in the hospice setting this is precisely what all staff, paid or unpaid, should be aiming for when listening to someone's concerns. This is difficult to achieve because we rarely pay each other such careful attention in our everyday relationships. Nevertheless, most see that offering advice about what to do is unhelpful and that when one is asked for factual or technical information, it is not too difficult to suggest a more appropriate person or offer to ask that person to speak to the resident or 'guest' at the day centre. (At Mount Edgcumbe Hospice people attending day care are referred to as 'guests'.) What is more difficult to learn when faced with a personal reflection, a fear or distressing thought is simply to encourage the person to go on talking and ways must be learned to facilitate this.

The difference between training of this kind for volunteers and for professionals is that the learning for volunteers remains at an essentially practical level – geared to their day-to-day tasks – whereas counsellors, psychologists and social workers would be expected to understand the theory which underpins the practical response and to be able to adapt it for use in other settings.

The original framework within which the CDH volunteer training was established came from the Telephone Helplines Association Guidelines for Good Practice which addresses selection, training and support and supervision as well as the important matters of confidentiality and equal opportunities. Because of the nature of the help required, volunteers were originally given substantial theoretical training on bereavement counselling. However, more recently, emphasis has shifted to experiential learning which includes working with a 'simulator' (a role-player who is a bereaved parent); like the hospice training, these sessions focus on learning to be 'other-centred', the main difference being that these volunteers need to learn enough to recognise signs of a complicated grief reaction; so when they think that they can detect signs of this, they can make use of the professional supervision which is at hand.

Training at most hospices and palliative care units is ongoing: not only in order to accommodate changes in the volunteer workforce or in council membership but because experienced volunteers recognise that they continue to learn, particularly in the area of developing interpersonal skills. Volunteers at Mount Edgcumbe, as members of staff, do have access to the hospice library and are encouraged to browse when they have time. There is always a day-workshop available for new volunteers either before they start or within one month and this is re-run about every three months, supplemented by 'one-off' sessions as demand indicates.

Support for volunteers can also include regular evening meetings roughly every two months – the content of these sessions is determined by what the volunteers need or want. Sometimes they want a speaker on an aspect of palliative care or volunteering, at other times they may want to share experiences or just hear an interesting speaker. Occasionally a few may wish to visit another hospice and they will then be asked to tell the group about it. Whatever the evening's event, the group always discusses ideas and feelings about their work and this is facilitated by the VSC. Other support is provided by the volunteer's line-manager and by the VSC on an individual basis when circumstances indicate a need for it. The CDH support is built-in through the presence of a supervisor during the telephone service hours and again, training and support are regarded as a continuing need.

Conclusion

There is already a variety of good practices established in working with volunteers in palliative care: the examples of practice described in this chapter have served to emphasise the very great value that volunteers bring to palliative care when they are selected and deployed appropriately and provided with good training and support. The issues raised included the need to keep equal opportunities to the fore and not rely simply on word of mouth in order to recruit; the importance of clarity in relation to role boundaries; a general emphasis in both the hospital and hospice settings on the importance of having written guidance on role, tasks and regulations, and the need for training to be volunteer-task related and for support to be provided by line-management 'on the job' as well as by means of group discussion.

It has become clear that the role of the volunteer manager is an exacting, responsible and skilled one, yet at the present time, no training or qualification is required. An increasing number of courses are now offered by the National Centre for Volunteering and some which do carry a qualification can be found at institutions of higher education. As the number of volunteers continues to increase, it seems both likely and desirable that an appropriate qualification will be required by organisations who employ people to manage volunteers. Meanwhile, the VSC's own professional organisation, the Association of Hospice Voluntary Service Co-ordinators, itself promotes good management practice, providing documentation for its members, training opportunities, conferences and regional meetings which target issues of volunteer management unique to the volunteer in palliative care. The enrichment of care in this field provided by volunteers has been very striking, encompassing as it does valued conversation with patients and their families and contributing to those activities which soothe and heal the spirit like music, aromatherapy and many others.

Resources

The Alder Centre Alder Hey Children's Hospital, Eaton Road, Liverpool L12 2AP

The Telephone Helplines Association 61 Gray's Inn Road, London WC1X 8LT Tel: 0171 242 0555

The Association of Hospice Voluntary Service Co-ordinators Secretary, Nightingale Macmillan Unit, 117a, London Road, Derby DE1 2QS

The National Centre for Volunteering Carriage Row, 183, Eversholt Street, London NW1 1BU

The National Association of Councils for Voluntary Service 3rd Floor, Arundel Court, 177 Arundel Street, Sheffield S1 2NU

9 Care management

'... community care is most appropriately regarded as a continuum extending from the individual receiving domiciliary support in their own home to those requiring an intensively supported residential or nursing home placement.'
(Alison Petch)

Care management is a means of delivering care in the community in which a budget-holder, in the form of a social services department or health authority, purchases services for people assessed as in need of health and social services. Needs defined as 'social' are means-tested, however, whereas needs defined as 'health' are not; in the absence of a clear national framework, this difference is a source of continual negotiation between the two organisations at local level. This also means that patterns of care management vary across the country.

The National Health Service and Community Care Act 1990, represented not only a changed attitude towards the institutional care, which had been standard provision for so many elderly people and for people with a mental or serious physical illness or a wide range of disability, but it envisaged shifts:

- From a service-led to a needs-based response
- From the local authority as provider to enabler of a mixed economy of provision
- From central to devolved budgets
- From a single service to multiple choice, and
- From a professionally determined to a user-led response. (Petch cited in Davies (ed.), 1997)

There is, on the face of it, a potential synthesis between these aims and the culture of palliative care which has developed in most of today's hospices, particularly in relation to needs-based and user-led responses. Because of cuts in central funding however, in many parts of the country the ill person's levels of incapacity must be quite severe in order to meet eligibility for service at all. Once eligibility has been established, then an assessment of needs is undertaken together with a financial assessment which determines the person's own contribution to their 'social' needs.

In palliative care the boundaries between 'social' and 'health' needs tend to become blurred and the assessment is frequently undertaken collaboratively by a district nurse and a social services care manager or community care assessor; the latter may or may not be a qualified social worker. From the service-user's point of view, whether or not their needs are assessed as 'health' or 'social' is of central importance, because of the financial implications. A further point of consequence to the recipient of social care from social services departments is that the care purchased for them is increasingly likely to be in the voluntary or private sector, chosen as the 'best value for money'. Some implications for these and related issues will be considered later.

Precisely how the needs of a seriously ill person are designated will depend upon a multi-professional assessment being made, usually by a district nurse and the local authority assessor or care manager, and often including the opinion of a consultant, not necessarily in palliative care. A decision must then be made as to what 'need' properly 'belongs' to which organisation. Such negotiations are of course set within the framework of local agreements between health authorities and social services departments but when both are experiencing severe cuts in central government funding, their assessors feel under pressure to resist accepting responsibility for any service which could arguably 'belong to' the other. The workload of the health professional, already under pressure, could be increased and for the care manager, money committed to one client could deprive another in equal need.

In order to alleviate some of these pressures, the National Council for Hospice and Specialist Palliative Care Services published in 1993 'Care in the Community for People who are Terminally Ill: Guidelines for Health Authorities and Social Services Departments'. The document cites the NHS Management Executive Circular EL(92)16 which defines the terminally ill as:

> ... those with an active and progressive disease for which curative treatment is not possible or not appropriate and death can reasonably be expected within twelve months. Such care and support may be provided in an in-patient, day or home setting, and should, wherever practicable, be available without regard to the individual's diagnosis.

The guidelines go on to emphasise the crucial point: 'The responsibility for financing the social and health elements of home care should be clearly established and agreed. The alternative could be conflict between health and social services authorities and a reduced choice and quality of life remaining for service users.'

In 1995, the Department of Health issued its own guidance: 'NHS responsibilities for meeting continuing care needs', emphasising that 'collaboration is crucial to ensuring the effective and integrated delivery of care' and that local eligibility criteria should be developed 'which will be used as the basis, in individual cases, for decisions about need for NHS funded care'. In relation to continuing care for terminally ill patients, one phrase in the DoH guidance has created much difficulty at the level of local agreement and that is that the NHS should continue to fund if the patient's 'prognosis is such that he or she is likely to die in the very near future'. The clearer guidance of a specified period had been replaced by a phrase which could be interpreted as meaning the next few days. Variations in local definition have been reported by our interviewees to be as great as two weeks to twelve months.

It is against this back-cloth that the following examples of practice have been chosen, as they reflect changes designed to improve the quality of care management within the bounds of local structures and policy and so far as possible, the guidance referred to above. The examples describe three different approaches to care management: from a voluntary hospice, an NHS-based palliative care unit and a local authority care management team.

Care management with negotiated delegation of health and social needs assessment to a hospice-employed social worker

Pat Mood, Senior Social Worker, Douglas Macmillan Hospice, Stoke-on-Trent

This is a 28-bed independent hospice, established in 1973 but still without a medical director/consultant in palliative care. The hospice also has a day-care unit for approximately 18 patients per day. The hospice serves a large industrial conurbation and surrounding rural areas; the area has been badly hit by the recession and pit closures.

The practice which has been developed is a system for identifying three categories for patients preparing for discharge home, according to their vulnerability and community care needs. The categories are:

1. Those whose needs have not changed and who therefore require only reinstatement of pre-admission services
2. Those who have slightly increased needs and are confident to await a visit from the social services assessor on their return home
3. Those who have complex needs or are anxious about the degree of care that they may need or those people whose needs indicate to the hospice

social worker that a process of negotiation between district nursing and social services is likely.

In the case of categories 1 and 2 above, the hospice social worker refers patients to the social services duty officer; in category 3, the assessment will be undertaken by the hospice social worker in collaboration with colleagues prior to the patient's discharge.

The introduction of this system was regarded as necessary both because of funding cuts to social services departments and the 'extreme uncertainty and lack of clarity following the community care legislation'. Patients were not assessed until after they had returned home and the distress which this caused seriously ill people was considered unacceptable by the hospice social work team. An additional concern was the increasingly cloudy area between district nursing and social services home care, the resolution of which could cause further delay in provision of service to the ill person.

The obstacles which had to be overcome in order to improve the situation for those about to be discharged from the hospice were a general resistance to change and a caution on the part of those involved in making the assessments to making a commitment which would inevitably mean that some other service users would experience delay in their own needs being assessed. Although the proposals had the initial effect of increasing tensions between district nursing and social services, once a set of criteria acceptable to everyone had been agreed, the arrangements were generally accepted as a helpful means of ensuring 'the best outcome for patients, their families and their carers'.

The key steps in realising the practice were as follows:

1. Discussing the problem and possible solutions within the social work team
2. Replicating this process at ward level and with the line-manager (in this case, the hospice matron)
3. Arranging a meeting with the district nurse manager and the social services group manager
4. Agreeing a formula (or protocol)
5. Informing others who needed to know of the proposed changes and further discussion to take into account their comments
6. Changing the practice to conform to the protocol
7. Monitoring and reviewing the implementation.

The most important basic principles underpinning the establishing of this kind of practice are identified as respecting the ill person's choice, ensuring support to families and carers and a commitment to providing the ill person with the best quality of life possible. Related objectives were minimising as much as possible the anxiety of social work and ward teams in a problematical area and facilitating recognition of roles and responsibilities of other professionals against a backdrop of scarce resources.

The resource implications for the hospice are slight and the benefits to the hospice social workers are that they no longer have to be present at home-based assessments nor do they have to argue the case for urgency on a case-by-case basis. Some time is also saved for the assessors, having now formally delegated the prioritising of complex needs to the hospice staff.

Care management in a hospital palliative care unit with emphasis on family meetings as part of the approach to needs assessment

Joyce Maccabee, Social Worker, Hayward House Palliative Care Unit, City Hospital, Nottingham

This is a 25-bed Macmillan Palliative Care Unit situated within the grounds of the City Hospital. The in-patient unit is primarily for pain and symptom control and respite care and the average length of stay is 2–3 weeks. Care for those in the last 3–4 weeks of life is offered to those who do not wish to go home, but the unpredictability of this phase together with the changing responsibilities of the health and social services can make this 'terminal' phase difficult to manage, when there is increasing pressure to admit new patients. The facilities include a day-care unit catering for 15 patients a day. The multi-professional staff are employed by the Trust, with the exception of the social worker who is a social services employee seconded to the Macmillan Palliative Care Unit.

The innovative practice which has been introduced into this unit is the holding of a meeting for family and/or key carers before a patient is discharged, where there are many people involved or where the discharge is likely to be 'complex'. The latter would arise if the ill person were judged to have a number of needs which would have to be met to ensure a safe discharge and to enhance resources at home if necessary; for instance, if the carer were themselves elderly or not in good health or the carer worked full-time and the ill person had restricted mobility. A family meeting is usually arranged on the recommendation of the weekly case conference at which each patient's needs are discussed by the multi-professional team. The ill person will already have talked to staff about their discharge from the unit and about any possible family meeting, so the relatives are not being empowered at the expense of the person who is ill. At this point, either the social worker or the primary nurse will contact the family member or a key person who will then ensure that others know. The family is seen first separately so that there is an opportunity to voice concerns and express hopes and fears which they might not feel able to do if the ill person were present at this stage. The staff attending the family meeting would be a registrar or senior house officer, the primary nurse or member of the appropriate nursing team and the social worker who chairs the meeting. Occasionally the occupational therapist or physiotherapist will attend but their main role comes into play at the home visit or when the home is assessed with regard to the physical needs of the patient. What is discussed at the family meeting will naturally vary according to the dynamic between members but essentially, the purpose is to enable members to explore their awareness of and their feelings about the condition of their relative. Questions will be answered by way of feedback from the multi-professional team's assessment following the case conference. The options of returning home, care in a nursing or residential home or care offered by a relative are then presented for consideration by the ill person and the family. The needs and wishes of the ill person, the resources of the family and their anxieties and concerns are further explored and support to them is also offered. The ill person is then included in whatever way seems right to them – he either joins the meeting or the group goes to his bed; or the family or particular family members join the ill person, with or without any staff. This process almost always clarifies the next step in the ill person's care.

The family meetings are seen as an essential component of holistic assessment and care in which the ill individual is seen as a part of the whole. It has been found that family cohesion is often strengthened by their engagement in the process. From the hospice's point of view, the family meeting is also an opportunity to effect maximum change with minimum staff input: all those whose understanding of the situation is necessary are present. The involvement of the whole family in the solution – whatever is finally decided – tends to increase commitment to it. (See Chapter 3 'Working with families'.)

The first key step in introducing the meetings was to establish the weekly multi-professional case conference chaired by the social worker. The second key step was to establish nursing 'teams' with a 'primary' nurse who would relate to a particular ill person and to their family. Commitment to introducing these new practices was undoubtedly strengthened by the position of the social worker who was seconded by social services as a care manager with knowledge of and direct access to a range of resources necessary to safe discharge. In establishing this kind of practice the social worker identifies three basic principles as relevant. The first is the approach of viewing the ill person as part of a family system, an understanding which affords both a fuller assessment and better supported package of care. The second principle is that of openness in communication – integral to the practice of family therapy from which the hospice-based family meeting draws its theoretical underpinning. Because the meeting involves doctors, nurses, social worker and occasionally other professionals, it models the general benefits of the principle in other aspects of collaborative work. The final principle is that of empowerment: in organisations staffed by professionals, service-users can often be excluded from information and feel that their own concerns and opinions are regarded as unimportant; the openness of family meetings can have an empowering effect.

Care management within a hospital-based local authority team in which one member has special responsibility for liaison with a local hospice

Pat Gardner, Care Manager, Kent Social Services

The context is an NHS Trust hospital serving a relatively urban part of a large county: the care management team members are seconded by social services and their role is to assess needs and purchase services for people leaving hospital or hospices in the area.

What follows is a different perspective on 'good practice' in care management from a social services-based care manager who has particular responsibility for accepting referrals from a local hospice. Also deployed in the hospice are social workers seconded by the same social services department but their role is defined strictly in terms of social work service provision within the hospice.

In this model, the care manager is part of a team serving hospitals in the area and she has, over the past two years, gradually become identified as the 'palliative care' specialist in the team and as the person who usually accepts 'cancer patient' referrals. As such, her remit includes servicing the local 20-bed independent hospice. In this Authority, when the care manager posts were introduced, they were seen as a different kind of job from social work and for some years the staffing policy view was that a social work qualification should not be the preferred one and this particular care manager's qualification is not in social work.

In order to establish herself within the hospice, the care manager gained agreement to attend the weekly nurses' meeting at which all the current patients' needs and wishes are discussed. This had two advantages: first, it facilitated mutual learning. The care manager learned about the impact of the illness and the various palliative treatments on patients and their families thus far; the nurses learned about working in response to the ill person's wishes, rather than to the professional's view of 'what the patient needs'.

Second, attendance at the nurses' meeting enabled the care manager to get some sense of who might want her services before she went on to the wards to let patients know who she was and what she might be able to offer. Some of the ill people might already know the care manager because she had met them at the oncology unit or they may have been referred for help earlier in the period of illness by their general practitioner. For the most part however, the contact would involve forming new relationships in order to establish whether or not the ill person wanted to be assessed for services on leaving the hospice. This care manager undertakes what she describes as 'gradual assessment', meaning that she takes her time, perhaps making several visits depending on how the ill person is feeling, and always ensuring that the person understands that a financial assessment will be involved. Occasionally, the ill person will decline services altogether on discovering that his home may have to be sold in order to pay for care, when his greatest wish is to leave something for his children to inherit. Whatever her view about the ill person's needs, the care manager in this situation has to accept his choice and 'walk away from it'.

If the ill person accepts an assessment, the care manager asks permission to contact his family. Within the framework of this model, the ill person is the 'client' and his family a potential resource for him. If members of the family need services as carers, then under the NHS and Community Care Act 1990, it would be the responsibility of the care manager to arrange for them to receive services. If however, the family has unresolved conflicts which are impacting on the ill person or there are indications that there might be a complicated grief reaction, the care manager would try to effect a referral to the hospice social workers. Otherwise, the purpose of the family contact is to explore the family members' willingness and ability to offer care or support to the ill person.

Self-care management schemes

A recent idea, currently being piloted in a number of local authorities, is that of self-care management in which the client takes on responsibility for choosing and purchasing his own services. In this model, an assessment of the client's needs is made and means-tested; a care-package is then costed, that is, at what it would cost the local authority to provide and this sum is paid into a 'care account' to be drawn on as and when the service-user needs help. Any unused amounts are periodically 'clawed back', leaving a small amount over to cover fluctuations in cost. Until the Community Care (Direct Payments) Act 1996 was introduced, money had to be paid through an independent agency which would then be responsible for providing services chosen by the client. This was thought to be preferable to provision by social services departments, as independent agencies could be more flexible in meeting fluctuating needs. Since the 1996 Act however, care managers have had three options: to use the services of an agency which receives a fee, to pay the money into an account administered by a carer, or, to set up an account for the client to draw on directly.

In Kent, the Medway Self-Care Management Pilot Project has been set up for disabled people who feel able to take on this level of self-sufficiency and a number of benefits and potential difficulties have already emerged. Because of the present financial constraints, the scheme only covers personal care, not domestic care. The direct payment model has proved to be of great benefit to some young disabled people who are able to do their own book-keeping efficiently. On the debit side, however, some individuals may be overwhelmed by the energy and administrative skills needed to take on not only the organisation of their own services but the problems inherent in becoming, in effect, an employer, and these would apply to the second option in which the carer receives the funds. The third option, in which an independent organisation is paid to act on the client's instructions within the agreed sum, seems to be the preferred one for many service-users, though it should be stressed that the pilot is ongoing and has yet to be evaluated.

These pilot projects were originally introduced to compensate for the closure of the government-sponsored Independent Living Fund which had been established for people with disabilities, but there is no reason why in theory it should not be used in palliative care. Women under 60 and men under 65 with, say, cancer or motor neurone disease might welcome the flexibility and speed with which their changing needs could be met. It may not be a helpful model however, for an ill person whose condition might be exacerbated by the stress of arranging and auditing their own services. Similar considerations would apply where the funds were paid to a carer.

Conclusion

The issues raised by these practitioners serve to underline the view that 'community care has a chameleon quality, susceptible to differential inter-pretation by different stakeholders' (Petch cited in Davies (ed.), 1997) and that there are many models of care management currently in use and constantly being adapted. As we have seen, however, the adaptations have resulted largely from the uneasy tension between managers struggling to cope with serious underfunding and professionals trying to offer the best possible quality of care in deteriorating circumstances.

As Petch has pointed out 'the defining feature of community care is its location at the junction of the health and social care divide' and as palliative care is by design concerned equally with the physical, psychological, social and spiritual dimensions of the ill person's well-being, this boundary becomes particularly difficult to deal with. Recently published research on care management either under-emphasises or overlooks the particular difficulties facing palliative care: it seems to be assumed that any person who is terminally ill must automatically fall within the remit of the NHS. The real progress which has been made in the control of pain and other symptoms when curative intervention has ceased, however, means that the period of palliative care can be substantial and varying in terms of the ill person's condition. An integrated package of health and social care is not only essential to the maintenance of life quality but it needs to be in place before the ill person is discharged from a hospital or hospice.

That the efficiency of hospital care is currently measured in part by its rate of through-put, has been accepted for some time by care managers or social workers based there and they have recognised that one of the skills they must acquire in this setting is to manage the tension between the hospital's need to clear beds and the ill person's need to know that they will be well cared for from the point of discharge. That some hospices increasingly see themselves as short-term symptom control facilities seems less widely understood. It is perhaps for this reason that in some parts of the country, care managers have not been pro-active in ensuring that systems are in place to meet the needs of the hospice residents. In this context, the first practice example is an interesting one: at an earlier point, the social worker here realised that some of the referrals were being treated as a priority by care managers very often by way of a visit on the day of the ill person's discharge. Not only was the person in question not necessarily regarded as a priority by the hospice multi-professional team, but to be faced with a strenuous care management needs and financial assessment interview, at a time when the ill person was likely to be feeling weak and vulnerable, was regarded by the social worker as potentially threatening to the person's condition. 'They were just sitting there with their calculators, deciding which of them would pay for what' was how one person had experienced the event.

Thus it was that the hospice social worker initiated discussions at middle-management level in the social services to find a better way of meeting the assessment and planning needs of those hospice residents who were ready for discharge. On becoming aware of the impact of current practice on the service users who were seriously ill, the manager concerned agreed at once that it had to be changed, underlining the benefits which can result from palliative care workers engaging with those in the statutory sector to produce better-quality service. The solution agreed upon did in fact increase the workload of the hospice social worker and her colleagues by requiring her to undertake the needs assessment of any person approaching discharge but she then knew that by evaluating someone as having 'complex' needs, a care manager would visit that person in the hospice before the anticipated discharge date and that they would have the benefit of direct and up-to-date information about the ill person from the hospice. Many other hospice social workers would have resisted such a solution as a matter of principle, seeing their involvement in care management in this way as a 'slippery slope' which would gradually change their role in the hospice. The hospice social worker's decision in the case cited was at one level a personal one, based on her own values and perception of what would most benefit the hospice patients. Although her colleagues in the statutory agencies may have shared both values and perceptions of need, it was the independence of the hospice which allowed it to make the changes necessary for the new system to flourish.

In the case of the Nottingham example, the social worker was employed in the statutory sector as a care manager and her role was therefore more restricted than her hospice colleague. In a sense, the families or carers were a potential resource for the patients who were ready to be discharged and the work undertaken with them was primarily to establish a soundly-based support network. In order for it to be secure, the social worker had, so far as possible, to meet their needs too, both as lay carers and as people who would later be bereaved. The good practice here was in integrating these needs within the role of care manager and in reducing where she could, the conflicting needs of carer and ill person.

Despite the great variation in interpretation of national policy, it is clear that the unifying factor in the above examples of practice is the value base from which the practitioners operate, looking always to respect the rights and needs of those they seek to help. Nevertheless, there remains an urgent need to standardise at least some of the continuing care criteria if care is not to remain a lottery dependent on geography; there is also an equal need for good palliative care practice to permeate into mainstream training for health and social service professionals.

10 Permeating the mainstream

> 'Why should the only minority who die of malignancies
> be singled out for deluxe dying?'
> (Douglas, 1991)

Despite its rapid expansion over the last three decades (Higginson, 1997), specialist palliative care can directly benefit only a relatively small number of ill or grieving people. It is therefore important that attention is paid to creative ways of educating and influencing the wider society in which people live and work. This chapter will examine ways in which palliative care can attempt to spread its principles, demonstrate its value and effectiveness and try to improve the extent to which the enormous variety of communities within that society acknowledge and resource the needs of those experiencing serious illness, loss and bereavement.

The widespread and long-standing use of volunteers in palliative care has been significant in spreading the word. It is interesting that it is only recently that the National Health Service has begun to exploit their potential in more creative ways (Department of Health, 1996). Volunteers represent the community from which ill people come and they return to it to influence its values. Volunteer staff also greatly extend the numbers of patients and families it is possible to support. For example, one social worker can supervise a team of ten volunteer bereavement counsellors, thus providing a considerable volume of service at a reasonable cost. The use of volunteers should not be a reason for reduced quality. Rigorous selection and appropriate training and supervision will allow volunteers to add considerably to the variety and scope of services to dying people and their families. The potential role of black and other minority ethnic volunteers in influencing knowledge of, and access to, specialist palliative care services has recently been acknowledged in recommendations that volunteers from these communities should be actively recruited and trained to assist health professionals in supporting patients and carers (National Council, 1995b).

197

Education has been one of the core objectives of the palliative care movement since the founding of St Christopher's Hospice by Dr Cicely Saunders in 1967. In 1959 in her document 'The Need' describing her vision for hospice care, Saunders wrote: 'There is a need for more teaching on this subject for students as well as nurses and a new centre for care should take some responsibility and try to help to fill this gap' (Du Boulay, 1994). Short training courses for doctors, nurses and other health care professionals both specialist and non-specialist have been joined by a variety of degrees and post-graduate qualifications (Smith 1994, 1996). More recently many units have offered training or support to other professionals who have to deal with the consequences of death; for example, working with the police on breaking bad news, accident and emergency department staff on managing sudden death and immediate bereavement care, teachers on responding to bereaved children in the classroom, clergy on taking funerals and funeral directors on emotional needs in bereavement.

Most trainers comment on the importance of including self-reflective exercises in course materials. Professionals' own experiences of loss or those losses they fear in the future are still prime inhibitors and unless understood can hinder or prevent skill acquisition. There is also increasing recognition of the value of training whole teams rather than a course of individuals from different organisations. St Christopher's Hospice has anecdotal evidence that inset days offering training to a whole school's staff of teachers have more impact on subsequent approaches to individual bereaved children, appropriate policy making and inclusion of death and loss in the curriculum. Training for teachers has been offered in age-related groups: nursery, primary and senior.

There have been some bold attempts to influence society to provide a more generally supportive environment for those experiencing loss and death. In Gloucestershire members of the palliative care team based at Gloucestershire Royal Hospital have set up 'Winstons Wish' (see Chapter 3) which offers a comprehensive county-wide service to all bereaved children aged 6 to 14, their families and schools (Winston's Wish, 1995). Political lobbying has also been effective, for example, the campaign waged by the Association of Hospice and Specialist Palliative Care Social Workers to change welfare benefit rules so that terminally ill people could claim the special Attendance Allowance more quickly. Professionals in palliative care have also been active in attempts to influence the euthanasia debate (National Council, 1993).

There is an active debate about how far specialist palliative care teams can or should attempt to offer direct care to those with non-malignancies (National Council, 1997b), driven in part by the requirement on health authorities to purchase appropriate care for all their residents, regardless of diagnosis. Many have criticised the palliative care movement for being slow to respond to the needs of the 'disadvantaged dying'. The government report 'The Principles and Provision of Palliative Care' published in 1992 demanded that palliative care be disseminated beyond cancer (SMAC/SNMAC). The needs of the elderly dying from other diseases have been highlighted. Seale and Cartwright (1994) revealed that up to 47 per cent of those over the age of 75 may spend the last year of their lives in residential nursing homes. Hospital support teams in acute settings have traditionally seen people suffering from a broader range of illnesses and have therefore offered an opportunity to improve the palliative care of many people including the elderly (Smith and Eve, 1994). However research has also indicated the failure of many geriatric services to deliver the palliation needed by elderly people who are documented as experiencing unnecessary distress in the last days of their life (Lloyd Williams, 1996).

The Calman–Hine report (Department of Health, 1995a) emphasises the importance of having palliative care services in all locations and that cancer patients can require palliative care services early in their illness, not just at the end. Seale (1991) points out that many of the chronically deteriorating conditions that have been resisted by specialist palliative care units, such as Alzheimer's disease, multiple sclerosis, respiratory or renal failure, are likely to present similar symptoms, and similar problems in bereavement, in both ill people and their families. The National Council for Hospice and Specialist Palliative Care Services has distinguished helpfully between the palliative approach: 'a vital and integral part of all clinical practice whatever the illness and its stage' and specialist palliative care services 'which use trained specialists in multi-professional teams to support dying persons, their carers and colleagues wherever they may be' (National Council, 1995a). However palliative care specialists clearly face the challenge of appropriately educating and supporting community services both directly and indirectly within the restraints of their own budgets and against competing demands.

Professionals in palliative care have much to learn from the strategies and value base of other charitable organisations whose consumer focus and skills in meeting the psychosocial needs of those earlier in their illnesses are highly relevant. The dilemmas about expanding service remit are also reflected in their practice. The remainder of this chapter will focus on the work of two cancer-based charitable organisations in both informing and supporting people with cancer, their families and their professional carers. It will also look at a hospice-based experiment to extend its services to individuals at an earlier stage in their cancer history and examine a project to extend training and support to nursing homes.

A service emphasising accessibility, self-help and user autonomy

Liz Urben, Self-Help and Support Service Manager, Cancerlink, London

Cancerlink is the national charity offering information and access to support, to anyone affected by cancer. Based in London, it maintains a database of local cancer self-help groups and a network of individual supporters throughout the UK and offers consultancy and training to people with cancer and to those who run cancer self-help groups.

Accessbility and flexibility

Cancerlink is trying to tackle the problem of health information and support failing to reach many of those who need it, working in collaboration with local community groups. It has made considerable efforts to actually put into practice a philosophy voiced by most health care professionals, stating in its publicity material that its mission is to provide 'support and information about cancer to everyone nationwide'.

Cancerlink runs networks of one-to-one supporters for people wanting to talk to someone in the same position. These include people with rare cancers, people from black or minority ethnic groups and lesbians. It runs a free telephone helpline for young people affected by cancer in conjunction with Macmillan Cancer Relief and runs an Asian cancer information line in Hindi, Bengali, Urdu, Punjabi and English. Cancerlink is working with other black community groups to raise awareness of screening issues among black and minority ethnic women. Its own wide range of booklets and fact sheets focusing on emotional and practical aspects of cancer are supplemented by videos and audio tape information in eight languages. Cancerlink's information leaflets stress confidentiality, an important reassurance often overlooked by other organisations: 'Our information lines do not user caller display equipment and we use line blocking on all outgoing calls.'

A particularly fascinating project that demonstrates an innovative way of responding to the needs of those who are geographically scattered, or who have rare cancers, is the telephone support group which brought together women from different parts of the UK who shared an experience of gynaecological cancer. (*Running a Telephone Cancer Support Group*, Cancerlink, 1994.) Cancerlink's commitment to collaboration is demonstrated by its joint work with the Black Cancer Care Project and its attempts to reach out to existing networks and groups, providing training, talks at conferences and back-up materials. Cancerlink also places a high priority on advocacy and influence with statutory services, collaborating with the Department of

Health on a project to improve the take-up of breast and cervical screening for women from minority ethnic communities and jointly producing a set of guidelines for commissioners on improving services.

Self-help, autonomy and control

Cancerlink has consciously attempted to deliver its services in a non-paternalistic way. It tries to ensure that as much control as possible stays with the person contacting the agency and to give them the information they want in a way that they can understand and use, with as wide a variety of perspectives as possible. Cancerlink's range of services, from individual networking to written materials, professional telephone advice and self-help groups, demonstrates its awareness that individuals need a variety of resources to choose from if their needs are to be met. Its mission statement speaks of focusing on 'the person rather than the cancer' and seeking 'to empower individuals, groups and health professionals by promoting self-help, good practice and equal access to services'.

Liz Urben stresses that the principles of palliative care are applicable at earlier stages for people with cancer and that quality of life issues are present from the time of diagnosis, through treatment until the time that the individual may be told there is no possibility of a cure. She recognises the inseparability of information and emotional support and emphasises the potential value of self-help groups in meeting these needs:

> Self-help groups can help to reduce the sense of isolation from family and friends ... People diagnosed with cancer can also feel powerless and experience loss of. control because of the focus on the cancer and its treatment. This feeling can be reinforced by healthcare settings in which patients are recipients of care from a system with which they are not familiar. [Urben, 1997]

The importance of social support as a way of reducing feelings of powerlessness has been increasingly recognised by professionals (Hitch, Fielding and Llewellyn, 1994).

Existing groups, or those considering starting a group, can register with the Cancerlink database, but they operate independently. For example, groups may be cancer specific or general, they may include volunteer services such as transport, run small information libraries, involve professionals or be entirely run by individuals with cancer. Almost all groups also offer support to families and friends and welcome the bereaved. People interested in starting a group are sent a starter pack and once registered receive booklets on issues to think about in self-help groups and information about Cancerlink's services. Cancerlink provides training and consultancy to those starting, facilitating or experiencing difficulties in running groups, whether they be individual group members or whole groups. There are currently over 500 groups registered in the UK. In 1992 Cancerlink published a survey called 'Celebrating Groups' which revealed that the majority of the groups are started by a person with cancer or a relative. Forty per cent have some professional involvement and one-third meet in a medical setting. A third of the groups had up to ten regular attendees and a third up to twenty. A member herself comments on the benefit of membership: 'I have learnt so much through this group in my search to conquer cancer. It has also been inspirational to meet another member who was given a few weeks to live, but is quite well now four years on ... The only negative aspect being the sadness felt when members actually die. Two friends passed away recently. It was very difficult for me but I am learning to live with this ...'

The consultancy service and training offered by Cancerlink attempts to help self-help groups overcome some of the weaknesses and disadvantages that often emerge in practice, for example, managing a disruptive or attention-seeking member, acknowledging the death of a member and dealing with the question of leadership. Many groups fall apart when the active founder member leaves, while in some groups the founder member does not want to share control and other members become frustrated and leave. Liz Urben points out that consultancy provided by an external agency such as Cancerlink can help a group manage these situations.

The basic courses offered by Cancerlink cover group facilitation, personal responses to cancer treatments, listening skills and issues around bereavement and loss. Additional training is also available on supportive therapies and topics that are perhaps less readily available elsewhere, although of major concern to those with cancer, for example, body image and sexuality, assertiveness skills, relaxation and visualisation. All Cancerlink courses are run in different parts of the country in order to improve access and take-up, and Liz Urben stresses the importance of addressing equal opportunities throughout training in planning both content and delivery.

Respect and a voice for consumers

Link Up is the quarterly magazine published by Cancerlink for consumers of cancer care. It contains a fascinating mixture of material, for example, personal views about the cancer experience, articles on how to complain, to find out about research, and to talk about death in self-support groups, as well as book reviews. The magazine is designed to give consumers a voice and focuses on cancer as a whole experience rather than just a medical one. It also acts as an exchange for passing on self-help groups' experiences and sharing good practice. Cancerlink tries to have only minimal editing of submitted articles and any rewriting involves the author. If you are thinking of visiting someone in hospital, listen to Rosa Auerbach first:

Do not use our loo. It may contain embarrassments that had to be hastily left when you came through the door. Do not turn on our television even if Sky does have 24 hours a day motor racing and you see no reason to miss any of it; our voices cannot compete. Moribund people seldom develop sudden new passions. So if we were bored witless by your cats, dogs, prize leeks before our illness, we still will be.

Also published are requests for support, for example, 'A lesbian with oral cancer would like to communicate by letter with a lesbian with oral cancer, other lesbians with cancer or women with oral cancer' (*Link-Up*, Autumn 1996).

Cancerlink's practice demonstrates its respect for the individual's right and ability to choose. It does not vet or validate groups but suggests to callers requesting information about local groups the questions that they might want to ask in choosing a group, advising them to consider how it is run, how it seems to respond to members' needs and so on. Cancerlink tries to ensure that dialogue between professionals and self-help groups is at a local level. When professionals phone with queries they are referred to the groups themselves. The determination to return responsibility and involvement to users is evident in Cancerlink's internal structure. Five elected group users are represented on the board of trustees and all groups can nominate and vote for them.

Cancerlink is also trying to influence the content and nature of public debate and understanding, compiling a list of people with personal experience of cancer who may be willing to talk to the media. Through *Link Up* they have advertised for people who might be willing to be interviewed, offering three clear assurances:

- Your name and telephone number would not be given to anyone without your permission. We would also contact you first and let you decide whether you wished to take part
- We would always brief you before an interview and run through the type of questions you could be asked and how you might like to answer them
- We would provide training and support if you felt you needed them.

The text also reveals Cancerlink's wish to empower those with cancer through the experience of being able to give as well as receive:

Everybody has a valuable experience and story to tell. In doing this you would be able to share your experience with others, perhaps reassure someone that they are not alone in what they are experiencing and help raise awareness of the range of support that is available. [*Link Up*, Autumn 1996]

A responsive organisation

The production of Cancerlink's training and information booklets is driven by the needs voiced by the consumers themselves. Thus a booklet on talking to children when an adult has cancer was the result of the huge number of telephone enquiries on this issue. All materials are pre-tested by the people for whom they are intended. Cancerlink often facilitates and helps to organise local training. For example, a cancer self-help group decided that their group would benefit from training on healing touch and Shiatsu as a number of members suffered from arthritis in addition to their cancer. Cancerlink provided and paid for a trainer and the result was a much appreciated day designed specifically for the needs of twelve local people. As a response to those who felt that very little information was aimed specifically at men, Cancerlink has produced a booklet entitled *Men and Cancer*, describing the experiences of a group of men of differing backgrounds and life styles. It looks at the impact of cancer from a male perspective, exploring men's experiences and feelings. Some of the men interviewed have cancer themselves: 'I do believe men should reach out more for help. I think we find it difficult to approach someone because society encourages us to be self reliant.' Some of them speak about caring for someone they love who has cancer: 'There were some very tender moments and she was able to accept my caring and loving in a way she hadn't before. She said she could love me to the edges. Nobody had ever said that to me before' (Cancerlink, 1996).

Challenges

Liz Urben comments on the continuing struggle to improve professional acceptance of self-help and support groups. Joint training and professional liaison with, and involvement in such groups, are ways of approaching this issue. Cancerlink also faces the difficulty of maintaining its 'hands off' approach whilst trying to be more pro-active about resolving some of the difficulties commonly faced by self-help groups. It is clear that baseline training is a key to group success. Cancerlink is exploring ways of improving take-up for training without imposing a particular group ethos or creating a series of clones following a pre-packaged model. Ideas include contacting those who do not attend training courses to find out why not, and actively following up groups who have requested a starter pack. There is also a question about whether Cancerlink should try to stimulate group development in order to achieve geographical cover.

An information and support service with a clear consumer focus

Catherine Dickens, Head of Cancer Information Service, BACUP (British Association of Cancer United Patients), London.

BACUP is a charitable organisation launched in 1985 by a doctor who herself had cancer. It offers a free telephone and postal information service, staffed by nurses with an oncology background. It is based in London and Glasgow where a personal counselling service is also available. It publishes a series of over 50 information booklets about aspects of cancer treatment, specific cancers and emotional issues.

A consumer focus – responding to changes in society

Cancer care and treatments have become more and more complex alongside a society (particularly the young) with an increasingly sophisticated attitude towards information and a media hungry for 'news', which sadly is often lacking in detail and perspective. The continued need for improved information for people with cancer is well documented (Audit Commission, 1993) and is emphasised in the recommendation of the Calman–Hine Report: 'Patients, families and carers should be given clear information and assistance in a form that they can understand about treatment options and outcomes available to them at all stages of treatment, from diagnosis onwards' (Department of Health, 1995a). BACUP explicitly attempts to address the power differential and communication gap that often exists between the medical professions and the person with cancer. Many health care professionals make assumptions. Some believe that the public start from a place of knowledge about the body and what can go wrong with it. Others maintain a paternalistic stance asserting that clinical detail is safer in the hands of the professional. Still more ignore completely issues that may not represent medical priorities but that individuals themselves are desperate to discuss: loss, sexuality, financial problems, difficulties in talking to friends and family.

Treatment options are bewildering: surgery is performed using different techniques, medication is ever more complex, new agents and drugs are constantly emerging, radiotherapy is delivered in different ways, hormones can be manipulated. Consumers of health services desperately need good information, yet they often lack access to appropriate experts and when they find them may discover that those experts have poor communication skills. In order to have a dialogue with professional carers and to make choices, individuals need a base of knowledge. However, they may not like to 'pester' those involved in their direct care: 'I don't want to upset the doctor.' Vicky Clement Jones, the founder of BACUP, wrote about her own experience of cancer, describing in particular her enormous need for information of all kinds and for that information to be repeated. Both she and the others with cancer that she met needed to get some kind of understanding of how chemotherapy worked in order to exert some control over the emotional experience of receiving it:

> For two weeks I was in tears every morning, plucking the lumps of hair from all over the bed clothes. Trying to lead a normal life while hair fell into my minestrone. Intellectually I understood what was happening, but emotionally it reinforced my feelings that I was losing a part of myself ... I eventually came up with a simple solution to deal with this, wearing a hair net in bed. I also wondered whether doctors and nurses looking after cancer patients had come across this problem, let alone a solution. I subsequently found most had not. [Clement-Jones, 1985]

Shorter stays in hospital mean that ill people need more access to self-directed sources of support. Expert advice and theoretical good practice in symptom control may not always translate easily to the home environment. The GP, who sees only a few people with cancer each year may not know the answers to all the complex technical questions around specific cancers and their treatment. In addition people are living longer with their cancers and the complex treatments themselves may well give rise to symptoms and effects that last well beyond the cessation of the treatment. People are effectively living with the consequences of their treatment as well as their cancers. They may also want information about clinical trials and what consent really implies. Questions are enormous and varied: 'What are the specific side effects of this treatment? Will it be painful? Am I going to die? How will I do the housework? What about the children?'

What information – who seeks it and how?

BACUP is based on the premise that appropriate information is what people want to know, given when they want to know it, in a way that can be understood. The efficacy of the telephone as a medium for conveying information about cancer has been well demonstrated (Venn et al., 1996; Rutter, 1987). Individuals contacting the BACUP telephone information service have already made a decision for themselves to do so. They control when they call and what they want to discuss. They are usually phoning from home, an environment where they feel more comfortable. They have anonymity and are not risking their relationship with someone involved in their direct care. The telephone also allows them to ask their questions alone. For example, a young woman with cancer may initially want to receive information about its impact on child bearing without the partner who supportively joined her at the hospital out-patient appointment. The telephone offers a permanently accessible opportunity to ask further questions rather than having to wait for the next month's appointment with the doctor. People with serious illnesses need time to process information and this time is not costed into the National Health Service system in the same way as, for example, surgery. For instance, fatigue represents a major problem for many people with cancer but it is hard for them to feel permission to talk about such a non-specific difficulty in a busy clinic (Fewell et al., 1996).

The Patient's Charter (Department of Health, 1991) declares as a standard that people should receive a clear explanation of any treatment proposed for them including information about risks and alternatives and that the information should also be available for relatives and friends should the patient so wish. However, the enormous number of calls to BACUP indicates a need for information about cancer that is not being met through the available National Health Service provisions. In 1995 BACUP distributed nearly a quarter of a million booklets and answered over 35,000 phone calls and 5,000 letters. Eighty-five per cent of those who contacted BACUP used the free phone line. In 1991 BACUP's information service was reviewed using a random sample of 406 callers selected over a ten-day period responding to a structured postal questionnaire. Of the 406 invited to take part, 282 responded. Interesting differences emerged between patients and relatives/friends in the predictors of emotional impact and satisfaction. The implications were that while patients are looking principally for information, relatives and friends are perhaps more concerned with reassurance. Such findings carry clear implications for the training of health care professionals. Overall the analysis indicated an overwhelming satisfaction (over 90 per cent) with both the information received and the nurses' communication skills (Venn et al., 1996).

Those providing the information: staff support

BACUP stresses that there is no substitute for information communicated within a personal context. The professional responding needs to know what the information means to the individual and to understand what it is that they want and need to know at the present time. An example of this would be helping a telephone enquirer to decide whether or not they are ready to read an information booklet which will cover much more information than the specific question they have been asking. It therefore follows that the nurses staffing BACUP's information service need to have a combination of expert knowledge (they have a minimum of five years' nursing experience, including three years in oncology and access to a comprehensive databank) and advanced communication and counselling skills.

Unpredictability is inherent in a telephone information service. BACUP is committed to maintaining the emotional health of staff so that they can continue to remain open to the enormous and often unexpected variety of questions and callers, many of whom are distressed.

Training

All staff have a six-and-a-half day initial training programme with a half-day follow-up. This covers counselling and communication skills. They attend annual weekend skills workshops on specialist areas that they themselves request, such as bereavement and talking to children. They attend fortnightly lectures from cancer specialists and patients' organisations. The importance of maintaining and developing skills beyond the induction training is stressed.

Supervision

All staff have group clinical supervision once a week with an external supervisor. The maximum group size is eight and this is seen as 'a safe place for restoration, support and critical reflection on practice'.

Handbook of practice

The handbook contains organisational objectives and group aims as well as guidelines on issues such as managing inappropriate telephone calls. It is available to all staff and updated with their suggestions and requests.

A partnership with health care professionals

It is vital to the success of BACUP's role as an information provider that it is accepted by health care professionals. BACUP actively aims to support the work of doctors and nurses who it sees as working under a variety of pressures. It tries to help callers to understand the health care system, and to involve them in choices about care, providing information about the existence of specialist clinics, alternative services and the roles of different professionals. For example, the exhausted carer of someone who is dying often also needs to be an expert manager of the large number of professionals who are visiting the dying individual. It can be confusing and overwhelming to know who to speak to about what. BACUP actively recruits the specialist expertise and support of senior and eminent medical colleagues in the preparation of their information booklets, the database and in training BACUP staff. In return the professionals get access to BACUP's knowledge of the difficulties faced by ill people and those close to them and the kind of information they are seeking.

Many aspects of cancer care and treatment are complex, controversial or of uncertain benefit. There has been a tendency to assume that where there is no hard information, where no one really knows the answer for sure, such information as is available should not be given to individuals with cancer as it might be too disturbing for a non-professional audience. BACUP has developed expertise in helping people to understand and cope with these uncertainties. It has worked together with health care professionals of all disciplines to publish papers on areas that are controversial and difficult for all. An outstanding example of this is its 'Statement on breast cancer, the pill and hormone replacement therapy', a review of the current literature circulated to all general practitioners (BACUP, 1995). BACUP co-operated with 50 other cancer organisations to produce *The Right to Know*, a statement of rights of people affected by cancer, for information and support, which also recommended standards for the Health Service to adopt in meeting these rights (BACUP, 1996). Other initiatives have been closer co-operation with occupational health resources in companies to try to influence the extent to which businesses support their employees with cancer (see Oliviere and Golding, 1996 for an interesting description of a workplace-based support group). BACUP is also in contact with pharmaceutical companies to maintain the latest product information and to return it with the questions and concerns of those who use the products.

The challenges

The majority of BACUP's callers are female, under the age of 60 and predominantly middle class. There are relatively few non-white enquiries (Slevin, 1988). The written materials it produces are more appropriate for an articulate audience with good reading skills. BACUP faces the challenge of attempting to maintain its focus and expertise whilst trying to respond more effectively to the needs of under-served populations. It is facing this challenge in the context of unmet need in its existing service. For every call that gets through, three get the engaged tone. BACUP is currently stressing the need for voluntary organisations to work together and to complement one another's skills and services. It offers its expertise to other organisations on a consultancy basis providing free access to its materials and allowing modifications where appropriate.

Initiatives to support nursing homes in providing palliative care

Mary Baines, Consultant Physician, St Christopher's Hospice and Consultant in Palliative Care to Croydon Community Health

Stella Hatcliffe, Quality Assurance Advisor and Wendy Lethem, Home Care Team Leader, St Christopher's Hospice, London

The need

Statistics show that an increasing percentage of elderly and dependent people are cared for in nursing homes (Seale, 1991). National Health Service reforms and demographic changes mean that the trend towards the care of more acute ill elderly people in nursing homes will continue. It is therefore vital that excellent palliative care should be available in all settings. The frail elderly with a relatively long prognosis and few major symptoms who can no longer manage at home should not generally be admitted to hospices. Most of them will receive better overall care by an admission to a nursing home in the first place, providing the nursing home can offer good palliative care. This requires good training and the readily available back-up of specialist domiciliary services. Short in-patient admissions to hospices (often with a fortnight's time limit) with a subsequent transfer to a nursing home when symptoms have improved, must be avoided. The emotional cost to the elderly person and their family of such transfers has been well documented by Maccabee (1994). For the majority of ill people it was a 'traumatic experience'. Both they and their families felt 'let down'.

The St Christopher's team had discovered that existing palliative care services were under-used by nursing homes despite the fact that they were the location of a significant proportion of cancer deaths in the area. In addition the local health authority had carried out a review of palliative care services which highlighted the need for training in nursing homes. The team was aware both of the need for support of any professional working with terminally ill people and that most generalist training barely scratched the surface of the emotional and physical needs of the terminally ill. Gibbs (1995) also remarks upon the enthusiasm of staff in nursing homes for meeting the palliative care needs of their residents, but emphasises their sense of isolation and anxiety about lack of post-basic education.

Meeting the need – a multi-faceted approach

It was clear that it would be necessary to provide support to nursing homes in several different ways in order to achieve and sustain change:

- Letters were sent to all matrons of nursing homes in the area reminding them of the existence of the telephone advisory service available from St Christopher's Hospice from 9 a.m. to 5 p.m. seven days a week. It was emphasised that this service, as well as all the others, was available for residents who were terminally ill whatever the diagnosis
- Nursing homes were offered the opportunity to refer a resident to the consultant in palliative care for a single visit, provided the GP's permission had been given. Alternatively they could request ongoing support from the home care team which would include clinical support from the nurses and doctor and specialist advice on emotional issues from the social worker. It was emphasised that the referral could be made by the matron (with the GP's permission) in order to make the service as easily accessible as possible
- Training in palliative care was offered to nursing staff in nursing homes. This could take the form of attendance at a central course or a single visit to an individual home when a whole staff group could be trained.

Issues in training

Various initiatives have been undertaken including collaborating with a private nursing home to provide a five-session course that could be purchased and attended by staff from other individual homes. Another initiative was achieved in collaboration with a neighbouring palliative care team. The course fee was sponsored by the health authority, as was preparation, teaching time and the provision of learning resources. Thirty places on the course were offered to senior nursing staff of the 16 nursing homes in the borough. The course consisted of four afternoons of training and had the following objectives:

1. To raise awareness of the support and advice available from specialist palliative care teams
2. To improve staff knowledge of symptom control
3. To explore specific issues of dealing with grief and loss in a residential community.

A variety of teaching strategies was used, including lectures, group work, case studies and role play. The importance of combining emotional issues and symptom control has been emphasised and evaluations demonstrated that this joint strategy was appreciated and valued by course members.

It was vital to make the course relevant to the issues and concerns of the course members, so their case examples were used throughout. Other important factors were understanding the particular differences for nursing homes due to the longer-term relationship staff had with their residents and residents' well-established relationships with one another. Equally, the trainers from the hospices had to be aware of the constraints of staff short-ages in nursing homes and the low ratio of trained to untrained staff. Course participants commented in their evaluations on the improvement in their knowledge of drugs and symptom control. There were other benefits too: 'I now find it easier to be more open about death with colleagues, residents and families.' 'I will now be looking more closely at the effect of the death on other residents and the staff.' The course increased the face-to-face contact between senior nursing home staff and local palliative care providers. Both palliative care teams have received referrals as a result. The next course will specifically target the ten homes not represented as the first course in an attempt to achieve overall coverage.

In conjunction with the practice described above, the social work depart-ment has also been delivering training to unqualified residential care staff focusing particularly on aspects of loss and communication with elderly residents. For example, they examine how other residents are told of the death of a fellow resident, what support they are offered and what involve-ment in the rituals of mourning is proposed, as well as ways of helping grieving partners or relatives. The two-day courses also examine the mecha-nisms through which nursing home staff can learn to support themselves and their colleagues as they cope with distressing situations. Clarke reports on a questionnaire completed by nine wardens of sheltered housing:

> None of their employing agencies provided any training for bereavement care. Not one had received any support from their agency in this area and seven felt they would appreciate more backup ... We all felt that we too needed to mourn, to be understood, supported and listened to, so that we in our turn could give our support, comfort and ears to our residents. [Clarke, 1996]

As Scrutton powerfully reminds us:

> There is a tendency for all of us to believe that bereavement in older people is a natural concomitant of the ageing process, and something that does not require help. Such an acceptance of loss in old age has led to a neglect of the support and counselling required by older people and their carers in situations that would clearly warrant such assistance with young people. [Scrutton, 1996]

Key requirements in establishing the practice

- Collect data including national and local statistics. Consult widely to obtain support. For example, the external support of the health authority and the involvement of the inspectorate both helped with funding and in raising general awareness of the importance of palliative care.

- Involve nursing homes themselves in planning both the services to be offered and the training to be delivered.
- The commitment of time and energy from the palliative care teams was needed over a period of months. Careful management and regular communication about the progress of the project was necessary to cope with the inevitable clash with the needs of direct patient care. The decision to train and support other professionals and to improve access to good palliative care demands more than lip service.
- Evaluation is vital. Data is being collected that indicates that specialist teams' input to nursing homes is increasing.
- Avoid a patronising attitude towards nursing home staff. Recognise their existing skills and the reality of the pressures in their particular environment. For example, the letter to matrons of nursing homes was worded thus: 'We are aware that nursing homes play an increasingly important role in the care of the elderly and dependent. Not surprisingly most residents and families would prefer them to stay in the nursing home during their terminal illness where they can be cared for by familiar staff.'
- Maintain regular contact with nursing homes after training. It is as vital to keep up the enthusiasm as it is to manage the bureaucracy that can feel like an obstacle. For example, before the letter was sent to matrons it had to be passed by community health, the inspector of nursing homes, the medical officer of health and through two meetings of nursing home owners.

A hospice-based short-term consultancy service

Frances Kraus, Principal Social Worker, St Christopher's Hospice, London

The consultancy service offers brief interventions to individuals with serious illness and their families/friends, previously excluded by a specialist hospice's referral criteria for full home care/in-patient services. The service is offered by social workers, doctors, nurses and physiotherapists, alone or in any combination. In practice, referrals, as was anticipated, have been mainly to the social work arm of the service. Clients are offered from one to five contacts with the opportunity for re-referral at a later stage or referral on for full home care or in-patient services.

Identifying the need

A small-scale survey of local general practitioners indicated that they were keen to have access to a service for people who were not appropriate for a full home care package. They highlighted the unmet emotional needs of individuals who were opposed to a referral to a hospice because they equated it with 'giving up and death'. They were also concerned about the needs of relatives who required someone with expertise in acute illness to talk to when the ill person himself was in denial. The GPs also spoke of their anxiety about the needs of people with complex bereavements where the experience and skill base of local bereavement services was often inadequate, and where access to local psychiatric/psychotherapy services involved long waiting lists and the consequent exacerbation of existing difficulties. The needs of bereaved children were mentioned and the wish to avoid stigmatising them with an appropriate 'psychiatric' label. Clinical staff at the hospice also hypothesised on the basis of their experience that some of the entrenched family communication difficulties picked up in terminal illness by the home care team could have benefited from much earlier counselling intervention. The consultancy service offered the opportunity to conduct a small experiment in meeting the palliative care needs of individuals earlier in their disease trajectory.

Establishing the service

A proposal was developed based on both the GPs' requests and information about unmet need derived from the hospice's telephone advisory service:

- Based on this data a charitable trust agreed to fund an additional social work post for three years
- All planning and development meetings have been multi-professional
- Evaluation was built in from the start of the project. One in five referrers and clients have been asked to complete a postal questionnaire
- The selection of the social worker was crucial to the success of the project. It was decided that the individual would need to be experienced in palliative care, familiar with the staff of the hospice, able to function alone, skilled at assessment and task-focused counselling and able to say no to inappropriate referrals. Consequently the post was appointed from the existing social work team at the hospice and the subsequent vacancy in the team was filled by a newcomer
- Publicity was initially low key to avoid a flood of referrals. All local GPs were circulated with a letter describing the consultancy service, a leaflet for giving to potential clients and a referral form
- All general practitioners get a closing report on the intervention.

What is good about the consultancy service?

Evaluations from both referrers and clients have been overwhelmingly positive. Emphasis has been placed on:

- Accessibility of the service
- Speed of response. Most clients are seen within days of a referral
- Value of expert advice and support which many referrers have commented has improved their own knowledge of a specialist area
- Many individuals' anxieties have been dispelled by a short-term counselling contract which has gently allowed them to accept a full home care package when appropriate
- Clients have appreciated a problem-centred approach that respects their autonomy.

Who has referred?

The bulk of referrals have come from general practitioners with a few from hospital consultants, teachers and clients themselves.

Who has used the service?

Clients have fallen into three main groups:

1. Patients with a serious illness but at an earlier stage than St Christopher's would usually accept, where there is a need for counselling. Case example: a 29-year-old woman with an unusual sarcoma in her head discovered during pregnancy. She was Irish, married to a Moroccan. They had two children aged 4 years and 6 months. Although her disease was incurable, she was currently undergoing treatment to contain the tumour and might well have a long prognosis. She received very little support from her husband but was fortunate to have a very supportive family who had been staying with her throughout. Her intention, not shared by her husband, was to return to Ireland. She appreciated the opportunity to talk to an outsider as feelings were polarised between her family and her husband.
2. Relatives of people with advanced disease who need to discuss their fears and anxieties often because the patient will not. Case example: a woman whose husband had advanced cancer and had left the family home very suddenly to live in a bachelor flat. The client was left with two teenage children and was unable to find out what was happening to her husband as rules of confidentiality precluded hospital staff from informing her. She needed intensive help and support with the process of accepting that her husband was unlikely to return and that she and

the children might well be excluded as he became less well. The children also needed to talk through their feelings of anger and rejection.

3. Complicated bereavement cases. Case example: a school referred a girl of 6 years after the child lost concentration in class and seemed 'very lost'. Her mother had died suddenly several months previously after falling down stairs. This child had woken up in the morning to be told that mummy was dead. She and her father were seen for five sessions. She needed to express her insecurity and anxiety about her surviving parent. The intervention concluded with the school report that she was working well in class, and father and daughter went on a successful holiday together.

Obstacles and difficulties

The service requires flexibility and often crosses accepted boundaries:

*   Some of the doctors and nurses involved have been more accustomed to firm referral criteria and were initially uneasy about the level of personal assessment required
*   Considerable inter-professional trust was required to accept the decision of a social worker that someone being seen under the service was less well and would need the fuller input of the home care service
*   The fact that the venue for most of the interventions was St Christopher's Hospice did not seem to prove a barrier to potential clients. Most of them were accustomed to out-patient appointments
*   How to publicise the service to general practitioners? They did not read publicity material. Word of mouth has proved most effective – this has been helped by the rule that every referral from whatever source requires the permission of the individual's GP. Attempts have also been made to publicise the service via district nurse bases
*   The isolation of the social worker, who is not defined as part of a multi-professional team and is working to a variety of referrers and a considerable client mix, many of whom are very needy. Good supervision is vital but the current postholder speaks of the rewards of extending the service to a wider section of the local community
*   Anxieties were initially expressed about the service's capacity to hold to a maximum of five sessions. In practice less than five per cent of cases have exceeded this and most of those have been working towards resolution as in bereavement. There have been relatively few inappropriate referrals, about one in six. Most of these have been cases that can be readily referred on, for example to social services departments, others are cases which reflect more about the worried referrer than the needs of the actual client.

What has been learnt?

1. Carers' needs for support are often unmet, particularly when the ill person is denying any need for help and the relative is left with unresolved fears and unanswered questions
2. There is a huge gap in the provision of easily accessible bereavement care for children and complex cases of adult bereavement. This is particularly true for work with whole families
3. Some very ill people need the opportunity for a gradual and non-threatening introduction to specialist palliative care services
4. Many people at an earlier stage in their illness lack access to counselling support
5. It is possible to effect considerable emotional change over short periods of time where the individual is highly motivated
6. The consultancy service is also used by professionals for access to counselling advice and consultation. Examples would be the local Macmillan nurses in hospital settings and a hospital consultant who requested the presence of the consultancy service social worker during a difficult interview: the bereaved wife of someone who had died from cancer was making a complaint.

Conclusion

The four descriptions of good practice in relating to and influencing the mainstream of care emphasise important themes: education and training, information giving and partnership with both service users and professional colleagues. Threaded throughout them are references to the increasing significance, in any service development, of issues of accessibility, flexibility in the mechanisms for delivering care and advice, respect for consumer choice and control and the necessity for appropriate evaluation. The indivisibility of needs for information and emotional support is stressed, underlining the requirement for health care professionals to possess not only expert knowledge but also the skills to communicate it, to focus on family and friends as well as the ill person.

Paradoxically, despite the growing emphasis on choice and an educated public, resource limitations means that such choices are inevitably restricted. Professionals in palliative care have a responsibility to ensure that their message is consistent with the 'products available'. For example, a generation has now been influenced to see 'hospice' as the place to achieve a 'good death', just as these hospices are increasingly defining, refining (and effectively rationing) what they consider to be appropriate referrals.

Given the huge number of potential service-users, economics and good sense dictate that coverage will only be achieved by effective advocacy and collaboration with existing organisations and networks and by the free and imaginative exchange of experience and information. There is evidence that better co-ordination of services can lead to substantial cost savings without loss of quality (Raftery et al., 1996). A paper (1996) by the National Council for Hospice and Specialist Palliative Care Services tackles the subject in *Working Together* which details local, regional and national inhibitions to good co-operation and makes suggestions for removing them. Despite the difficulties of competition for example for charitable funds and NHS contracts, it is clear that Bosanquet is right to declare that 'new alliances are needed for shared care if the full promise of palliative care is to be realised' (Bosanquet, 1997).

The dilemma of when palliative care should start and to whom it should be offered will remain a key debate for specialists in the field. The vision of universal access to good palliative care regardless of diagnosis or setting will require a major commitment of time, energy and physical resources on the part of specialist teams. Effective education demands a collaborative and flexible approach that respects the needs and constraints of differing professionals rather than the imposition of internally accepted service standards and techniques of delivery. Any such training will be rendered ineffective if it neglects the requirement to examine and improve the personal support mechanisms of professional carers. The efforts of a variety of voluntary organisations and lobby groups mean that health care professionals will increasingly be presented with the challenge of creatively educated consumers, some of whom may know more than the professionals themselves. Working with such consumers will mean really engaging in the struggles and rewards of the dialogue that has for so long been proclaimed as a vital component in effective health care.

Resources

BACUP 3 Bath Place, Rivington Street, London EC2A 3JR. Tel: 0171 696 9003

Cancerlink 11–21 Northdown Street, London N1 9BN. Tel: 0171 833 2818

Help the Hospices 34–44 Britannia Street, London WC1X 9JG. Tel: 0171 278 5668
A grant-giving charity which helps to organise and fund education and training opportunities for providers of palliative care

Hospice Information Service, St Christopher's Hospice 51–59 Lawrie Park Road, London SE26 6DZ. Tel: 0181 778 9252. Acts as a world-wide link to encourage sharing of information and experience amongst those involved in palliative care

Macmillan Cancer Relief Anchor House, 15–19 Britten Street, London SW3 3TZ. Tel: 0171 351 7811. Supports and develops services to provide specialist care for people with cancer at every stage of their illness. Also provides financial help through patient grants

Marie Curie Cancer Care 28 Belgrave Square, London SW1X 8QG. Tel: 0171 235 3325. Provides eleven centres in the UK, over 6,000 Marie Curie nurses to care for people in their own homes, a Research Institute and an Education Department for health professionals

National Council for Hospice and Specialist Palliative Care Services 7th Floor, 1 Great Cumberland Place, London W1H 7AL. Tel: 0171 269 4550. Acts as the co-ordinating and representative organisation for hospice and palliative care services in England, Wales and Northern Ireland

Conclusion

In this book we have sought to capture examples of good and innovative practice in psychosocial palliative care. The first chapter attempts to encapsulate the experience of being a dying patient or a carer, using four case studies in which the individuals speak for themselves about their own perceptions of care. Each subsequent chapter has been based on recorded interviews with practitioners who have described and commented on their work.

We are aware that there are other examples of excellent and innovative practice in parts of the United Kingdom which were less accessible to us, but despite this restriction, believe that the experiences described here will have provided valuable ideas and models of practice.

Several themes have recurred, the most evident being the constant reference by practitioners to their professional values. These included respect for individuality, patient autonomy and empowerment, enhancing the quality of life and equal opportunities both for patients in accessing services and for staff and volunteers in the workplace. The extensive contribution made by volunteers to palliative care has also become apparent in several chapters other than the one devoted to that particular topic. Another recurring theme has been multi-professional teamwork, in which good practice sees the virtual abandonment of the traditional status of one profession over another and a mutual respect for the validity of each discipline's knowledge and skill. The most striking partnership, however, has been that between the professional and the ill person, emphasised in every example of practice.

These accounts have numerous implications for practice in the future. One of the most important publications relevant to palliative care to come from government in recent years is the Calman–Hine Report, *A Policy*

Framework for Commissioning Cancer Services: a Report by the Expert Advisory Group on Cancer to the Chief Medical Officers of England and Wales (Department of Health, 1995). One of its key recommendations, the establishing of cancer centres across the country, is now being implemented, and training programmes and research projects will undoubtedly be attached to them, providing opportunities for developments in psychosocial aspects of palliative care as well as medical interventions and physical care. It would be a retrograde step in palliative care, however, if the treatment of cancer were to become the sole focus for government-supported innovations in the field, when we have seen hospices and specialist palliative care services extend their work in recent years to people with other illnesses which are unresponsive to treatment – especially those with the more chronic and longer-term conditions.

There is also a debate about whether or not the particular knowledge and skills of palliative care should be confined within specialist organisations who may then offer consultancy to other groups (which would certainly fit well with the present 'market' culture) or whether the expertise should be passed on through the qualifying training programmes of those engaged in the work. In particular, there is certain to be a further burgeoning of private nursing and care homes: demographic projections alone make this inevitable and great numbers of elderly people will die in these facilities. Good palliative care skills will much enhance the end of life for those people and it is argued that an urgent training focus should be in that sector.

A further government initiative is needed to resolve the anomalies in continuing care in which, at worst, it is possible for a person to die without the appropriate services because of delays at local level in determining which agency is financially responsible for their provision. This is one aspect of palliative care which would benefit greatly from the setting of national standards and at the time of writing, interested groups are pressing hard for such changes.

For practitioners, two issues in particular have emerged which we believe will need addressing in the future. One is to develop a greater sensitisation to the differing experiences of men and women and of different ethnic communities so that the needs of specific groups are not lost within a trend to standardise services in order to achieve 'value for money'. The second issue which is not only evidenced in the first chapter but is implicit in most of the others, is a continuing need to increase patient and carer involvement and consultation in shaping policy and services. In particular, we need to learn the best ways to engage them in providing feedback and not assume that because someone is dying, they are unable or unwilling to contribute to improvements in care. How do we meet the challenges of 'working together' and 'patient partnership' and make these concepts real?

Good practice in palliative care also involves staff in evolving their own set of survival skills. As Vachon reminds us, '... it takes a "total person" to respond day after day to the "total needs" of other people' (Vachon, 1995). It is essential that, in order to remain 'in balance', professionals have access to opportunities for support, supervision and consultation, as well as permission to be 'off duty'. An ongoing challenge for palliative care is to go on creating imaginative support systems, both formal structures and individual strategies. Further studies are needed to guide us in finding those supports which are experienced as most sustaining by those who engage in this emotionally demanding work.

Finally, there are clear indications from our interviews with patients, carers and professionals that future research in palliative care needs to focus as much on psychosocial aspects as on technological developments. It is often easier to fund the latter because of commercial interests but as Sheldon (1997) reminds us: 'Saunders' vision was to maintain a holistic and humane approach in partnership with the best of modern therapeutic care, and research is certainly necessary if this fruitful tension is to continue.'

References

Abeles, M., Oliviere, D. and Pyke, M. (1995) 'Groups with a difference', *Bereavement Care* **14**(2): 14–16.

Addington-Hall, J. and McCarthy, M. (1995) 'Dying from cancer: results of a national population-based investigation', *Palliative Medicine* **9**(4): 295–305.

Anderson, G. R. (1995) 'Children and HIV: orphans and victims' in Doka, K. J. (ed.) *Children Mourning, Mourning Children*, Washington: Hospice Foundation of America.

Audit Commission (1993) *What Seems to be the Matter: Communication between Hospitals and Patients*, London: HMSO.

Auerbach, Rosa (1996) 'Cancer ward – A visitor's guide', *Link Up* **45**(14), London: Cancerlink.

BACUP (1995) *Breast Cancer, the Pill and Hormone Replacement Therapy: Statement Series*, No. 1, November, London: BACUP.

BACUP (1996) *The Right to Know*, London: BACUP.

Baulkwill, J. and Wood, C. (1994) 'Groupwork with bereaved children', *European Journal of Palliative Care*, **1**(3): 113–115.

Benson, J. and Britten, N. (1996) 'Respecting the autonomy of cancer patients when talking with their families', *British Medical Journal*, **313**(21 September): 699–700.

Bierhals, A. J. et al. (1996) 'Gender differences in complicated grief among the elderly', *Omega*, **32**: 303–317.

Black, D. (1994) 'Psychological reactions to life-threatening and terminal illnesses and bereavement' in Rutter, M., Taylor, E. and Hersov, L. (eds) *Child and Adolescent Psychiatry. Modern Approaches*, 3rd edn, Oxford: Blackwell.

Black, D. and Young, B. (1995) 'Bereaved children: risk and preventive intervention' in Raphael, B. and Burrows, G. (eds), *Handbook of Studies on Preventive Psychiatry*, Amsterdam: Elsevier.

Bosanquet, N. (1997) 'New challenge for palliative care', *British Medical Journal*, **314**(3 May): 1294.

Bottomley, A. (1997) 'Cancer support groups – are they effective?', *European Journal of Cancer Care*, **6**: 11–17.

Bourne, S. (1997) Personal communication.

Brandes, D. and Phillips, H. (1990) *Gamester's Handbook*, Cheltenham: Stanley Thornes.

Broadbent, M. et al. (1990) 'Bereavement Groups', *Bereavement Care*, **9**(2): 14–16.

Brobant, S. (1992) 'Grieving Men: thoughts feelings and behaviours following death of wives', *Hospice Journal*, **8**: 33–47.

Bromberg, M. H. and Higginson, I. (1996) 'Bereavement follow-up. What do palliative care support teams actually do?', *Journal of Palliative Care*, **12**(1): 12–17.

Brown, H. C. (1997a) *Social Work and Sexuality. Working with Lesbians and Gay Men*, Basingstoke: Macmillan.

Brown, H. C. (1997b) Personal communication.

Burnell, A. (1994) 'Working with bereaved fathers', *Bereavement Care*, **13**(3): 28–30.

Byrne, G. J. (1996) 'A longitudinal study of bereavement phenomena in recently widowed elderly men', *Psycholmed*, **24**(2): 411–421.

Cancerlink (1993) *Body Image, Sexuality and Cancer*, 3rd edn, London: Cancerlink.

Cancerlink (1994) Rosenfield, M. and Urben, L., *Running a Telephone Cancer Support Group*, London: Cancerlink.

Cancerlink (1995a) *Close Relationships and Cancer*, London: Cancerlink.

Cancerlink (1995b) *Guidelines for Commissioners and Providers of Cancer Care. Towards Better Services for Black and Minority Ethnic People with Cancer*, London: Cancerlink.

Cancerlink (1996), *Men and Cancer*, London: Cancerlink.

Capone, M. A. et al. (1980) 'Psychosocial rehabilitation of gynaecologic oncology patients', *Archives of Physical Medicine and Rehabilitation*, **61**: 128–132.

Carter, B. and McGoldrick, M. (1988) 'Overview: the changing family life cycle' in Carter, B. and McGoldrick, M. (eds) *The Changing Family Life Cycle: A Framework for Family Therapy*, New York: Gardner Press, 3–28.

Clarke, J. (1996) 'After a death in sheltered housing: The warden's job', *Bereavement Care*, **15**(3): 30–1.

Clement-Jones, V. (1985) 'Cancer and beyond: the formation of BACUP', *British Medical Journal*, **291**: 1021–1023.

Congress, E. (1994) 'The use of culturalagrams to assess and empower culturally diverse families', *Journal of Contemporary Human Services*, **46**: 531–540.

Counsel & Care (1995) *Last Rights. A Study on how Death and Dying are Handled in Nursing Homes*, London: Counsel & Care.

Crowther, M. E., Corney, R. H. and Shepherd, J. H. (1994) 'Psychosexual implications of gynaecological cancer', *British Medical Journal*, **308**(2 April): 869–870.

Davies, M. (1997) (ed.) *The Blackwell Companion to Social Work*, Oxford: Blackwell Publishing Ltd.

Dean, R. A. (1997) 'Humour and laughter in palliative care', *Journal of Palliative Care*, **13**(1): 34–39.

Department of Health (1989) *Caring for people – Community Care in the Next Decade and Beyond*, Cm. 849, London: HMSO.

Department of Health (1991) *The Patient's Charter*, 51–1003 10/91 C5,000, London: HMSO.

Department of Health (1995a) *A Policy Framework for Commissioning Cancer Services (The Calman–Hine Report)*, London: Department of Health.

Department of Health (1995b) *NHS Responsibilities for Meeting Continuing Care Needs: letter guidance on HSG (95) 8 and LAC (95) 5*, London: Department of Health.

Department of Health (1996) *Making a Difference: Strengthening Volunteering in the NHS*, London: NHS Executive Department of Health.

Department of Health Social Services Inspectorate (1996) *Working alongside volunteers. Promoting the role of volunteers in community care*, London: Department of Health.

Doel, M. (1994) 'Task-centred work', in Hanvey, C. and Philpot T. (eds) *Practising Social Work*, London: Routledge.

Douglas, C. (1991) 'For all the saints', *British Medical Journal*, **304**: 579.

Doyle, D. (1996) 'Breaking bad news: starting palliative care', Lecture reported in *Journal of the Royal Society of Medicine*: **89**(10): 590–591.

Du Boulay, S. (1994) *Cicely Saunders*, London: Hodder and Stoughton.

Dunn, E. V. et al. (eds) (1994) *Disseminating Research/Changing Practice*, London: Sage.

Dwivedi, K. N. (ed.) (1993) *Group Work with Children and Adolescents – A Handbook*, London: Jessica Kingsley.

Earnshaw-Smith, E. and Yorkstone, P. (1986) *Setting up and Running a Bereavement Service* London: St Christopher's Hospice.

Eastaugh, A. N. (1996) 'Approaches to palliative care by primary health care teams', *Journal of Palliative Care*, **12**(4): 47–50.

Elliott, B. (1979) 'Sexual needs of those whose partner has died', *Bereavement Care*, **16**(1): 2–5.

Fallowfield, L. (1992) 'The quality of life: sexual function and body image following cancer therapy', *Cancer Topics*, **9**(2): 20–21.

Fewell, B. R. et al. (1996) ' "Bone Tired" The experience of fatigue and its impact on quality of life', *Oncology Nursing Forum*, **23**(10): 1539–47.

Field, D., Hockey, J. and Small, N. (1997) 'Making sense of difference. Death, gender and ethnicity in modern Britain' in Field, D., Hockey, J. and Small, N. (eds) *Death, Gender and Ethnicity*, London: Routledge.

Frank, A. (1991) *At the Will of the Body: Reflections of Illness*, Boston: Houghton Mifflin.

Geissler, E. M. (1994) *Cultural Assessment*, Pocket Guide, St Louis, USA: Mosby.

Gelcer, E. (1983) 'Mourning is a family affair', *Family Processes*, **22**(4): Dec. 1983.

Gibbs, G. (1995) 'Nurses in private nursing homes: a study of their knowledge and attitudes to pain management in palliative care', *Palliative Medicine*, **9**(3): 245–253.

Gill, P. (1997) 'Male sexual problems in palliative care', *Palliative Care Today*, **5**(4): 46–47.

Gilley, J. (1988) 'Intimacy and terminal care', *Journal of the Royal College of General Practitioners*, **38**: 121–122.

Green, J. (1991) Vol. 1 (1993) Vol. 2, *Death with Dignity. Meeting the Spiritual Needs of Patients in a Multi-cultural Society*, A Nursing Times Publication, London: Macmillan Magazines Ltd.

Guardian (1994) 'Pupils rely on friends for facts of life', 28 March 1994, *The Guardian*, London.

Gunaratnam, Y. (1993) *Health and Race Checklist*, London: King's Fund.

Hagemeister, A. and Rosenblatt, P. (1997) 'Grief and the sexual relationship of couples who have experienced a child's death', *Death Studies*, **21**: 231–252.

Hall, J. and Kirschling, J. M. (1990) 'A conceptual framework for caring for families of hospice patients' in Kirschling, J. M. (ed.) *Family-based Palliative Care*, New York: Haworth.

Haroon-Iqbal, H. et al. (1995) 'Palliative care services for ethnic groups in Leicester', *International Journal of Palliative Nursing*, **1**:(2).

Haworth, M. et al. (1997) 'Asian interpreters and palliative care. Research Abstracts', *Palliative Medicine*, **11**: 77.

Heegaard, Marge (1988) *Facilitator Guide for 'When Someone Very Special Dies'*, Minneapolis, USA: Woodland Press.

Hicks, C. and Hennessy, D. (1997) 'Mixed messages in nursing research: their contribution to the persisting hiatus between evidence and practice', *Journal of Advanced Nursing*, **25**(3): 595–601.

Hicks, C. et al. (1996) 'Investigating attitudes to research in primary health care teams', *Journal of Advanced Nursing*, **24**(5): 1033–41.

Higginson, I. (1993) 'Palliative Care: A review of past, changes and future trends', *Journal of Public Health Medicine*, **15**(1): 3–8.

Higginson, I. (1997) 'Palliative and terminal care' in Stevens, A. and Raftery, J. (eds) *Health care needs assessment*, Oxford: Radcliffe Medical Press.

Higginson, I., Hearn, J. and Webb, D. (1996) 'Audit in palliative care: does practice change?', *European Journal of Cancer Care*, **5**: 233–236.

Hitch, P. J., Fielding, R. G. and Llewelyn, S. P. (1994) 'Effectiveness of self help and support groups for cancer patients: a review', *Psychology and Health*, **9**: 437–448.

Hughes, M. (1995) *Bereavement and Support – Healing in a Group Environment*, Washington: Taylor & Francis.

Institute of Cancer Research, Royal Marsden NHS Trust, Cancer Relief Macmillan Fund (1995) *Living with Breathlessness*, London: Centre for Cancer and Palliative Care, Institute of Cancer Research.

Jaffe, L. (1979) 'Sexual problems of the terminally ill' in Pritchard, E. R. et al. (eds) *Home Care Living with Dying*, New York: Columbia University Press.

Kalish, R. A. (1985) *Death, Grief and Caring Relationships*, 2nd edn, California: Brooks Cole.

Kirschling, J. M. (ed.) (1990) *Family-based Palliative Care*, New York: Haworth.

Kraus, F. (1996) 'Confronting the reality of terminal illness', *European Journal of Palliative Care*, **3**(4): 167–170.

Lamerton, R. (1986) *East End Doc*, Cambridge: Lutterworth.

Littlewood, J. C. (1991) 'Gender differences in parental coping following their child's death', *British J. Guidance and Counselling*, **19**(2): 139–149.

Livesey, P. (1996) *The GP Consultation*, Oxford: Butterworth-Heinemann.

Lloyd Williams, M. (1996) 'A survey of palliative care given to patients with end stage dementia' [Abstract], *Palliative Medicine*, **10**(1): 63.

Lomas, J. and Haynes, R. B. (1989) 'A Taxonomy and critical review of tested strategies for the application of clinical practice recommendations: from 'official' to 'individual' clinical policy', *American Journal of Preventive Medicine 1988*, **4**(4 S): 77–95.

Lothian Racial Equality Council (1992) *Religions and Cultures. A guide to patients' beliefs and customs for health service staff*, Edinburgh: LREC.

Lukas, S. (1993) *Where to Start and What to Ask. An Assessment Handbook*, London: Norton.

Lum, P. (1992) *Social Work Practice and People of Color: a Process and Stage Approach*, 2nd edn, Pacific Grove, CA: Brooks Cole.

McGoldrick, M. and Gerson, R. (1985) *Genograms in Family Assessment*, New York: Norton.

McGough, R. (1990) 'Today is not the day for adultery' in *Blazing Fruit: Selected Poems*, London: Penguin.

Maccabee, J. (1994), 'The effect of transfer from a palliative care unit to nursing homes – are patients' and relatives' needs met?', *Palliative Medicine*, 8(3): 211–214.

Malatesta, V., Chambless, D. et al. (1988) 'Widowhood, sexuality and ageing', *Sexual and Marital Therapy*, 14(1): 49–62.

Monroe, B. (1993a) 'Psychosocial dimensions of palliation' in Saunders, C. and Sykes, N. (eds). *The Management of Terminal Malignant Disease*, 3rd edn, London: Edward Arnold.

Monroe, B. (1993b) 'Social work and palliative care' in Doyle, D., Hanks, G. and Macdonald, N. (eds) *Oxford Textbook of Palliative Medicine*, Oxford: Oxford University Press.

Monroe, B. (1997), *Facilitated Groups for People with Terminal Illness*, Proceedings of IV Congress of the European Association for Palliative Care, 6–9 December 1995, Barcelona.

National Association of Bereavement Services (1996) *Bereavement Care – Developing a Quality Service*, London: National Association of Bereavement Services.

National Council for Hospice and Specialist Palliative Care Services (1993) *Key Ethical Issues in Palliative Care: Evidence to House of Lords Select Committee on Medical Ethics. Occasional Paper No. 3*, July 1993, London: National Council.

National Council for Hospice and Specialist Palliative Care Services (1993) *Care in the Community for People who are Terminally Ill: Guidelines for Health Authorities and Social Services Departments*, London: National Council.

National Council for Hospice and Specialist Palliative Care Services (1995a) *Specialist Palliative Care: a Statement of Definitions. Occasional Paper No. 8*, October 1995, London: National Council.

National Council for Hospice and Specialist Palliative Care Services (1995b), Hill, D. and Penso, D., *Opening Doors: Improving Access to Hospice and Specialist Palliative Care Services by Members of the Black and Ethnic Minority Communities. Occasional Paper No. 7*, January 1995, London: National Council.

National Council for Hospice and Specialist Palliative Care Services (1996). *Working Together*, London: National Council.

National Council for Hospice and Specialist Palliative Care Services (1997a), *Voluntary Euthanasia: The Council's View*, July 1997, London: National Council.

National Council for Hospice and Specialist Palliative Care Services (1997b) Doyle, D., *Dilemmas and Directions: The future of palliative care: Occasional Paper II*, February 1997, London: National Council.

National Council for Hospice and Specialist Palliative Care Services (1997c) *Feeling Better: psychosocial care in specialist palliative care. A discussion paper. Occasional Paper 13*, August 1997, London: National Council.

Neuberger, J. (1994) *Caring for Dying People of Different Faiths*, 2nd edn, London: Mosby.

Neville, R. (1995) 'Making memory stores with children and families affected by HIV' in Smith, S. and Pennells, M. (eds) *Interventions with Bereaved Children*, London: Kingsley.

Odier, C. (1996) *Lecture, Diplôme Universitaire de Soins Palliatifs*, Université Catholique de Lille, April 1996.

Oliviere, D. (1993) 'Cross-cultural principles of care' in Saunders, C. and Sykes, N. (eds) *The Management of Terminal Malignant Disease*, 3rd edn, London: Edward Arnold.

Oliviere, D. and Golding, V. (1996) 'Coping at Work', *Link Up*, **46**: 11–13, London: Cancerlink.

O'Neill, J. (1994) 'Ethnic minorities – neglected by palliative care providers', *Journal of Cancer Care*, **3**: 2145–220.

Oppenheim, L. (1998) Personal communication.

Parkes, C. M. (1975) 'The emotional impact of cancer on patients and their families', *Journal of Oncology and Laryngology*, **89**: 1271–1279.

Parkes, C. M., (1966) *Bereavement: Studies of Grief in Adult Life*, 3rd edn, London: Tavistock.

Parkes, C. M., Laungani, P. and Young, W. (eds) (1997) *Death and Bereavement Across Cultures*, London: Routledge.

Parkes, C. M., Relf, M. and Couldrick, A. (1996) *Counselling in Terminal Care and Bereavement*, Leicester: British Psychological Society.

Payne, S. and Relf, M. (1994) 'The assessment of need for bereavement follow-up in palliative and hospice care', *Palliative Medicine*, **8**:291–297.

Peabody, F. W. (1927) 'The care of the patient', *Journal of the American Medical Association*, **88**:877–882.

Phelan, M. and Pankman, S. (1995) 'Working with an Interpreter', *British Medical Journal*, **311**: 555–557.

Poorman, S. (1983) 'Human sexuality and nursing practice' in Stuart, G. S. and Sundeen, S. J. (eds) *Principles and Practice of Psychiatric Nursing*, 2nd edn, Missouri: Mosby.

Raftery, J. P. et al. (1996) 'A randomized controlled trial of the cost effectiveness of a district co-ordinating service for terminally ill cancer patients', *Palliative Medicine*, **10**(2): 151–61.

Randall, F. and Downie, R. S. (1996) *Palliative Care Ethics. A Good Companion*, Oxford: Oxford University Press.

Raphael, B. (1982) *The Anatomy of Grief*, New York: Basic Books.

Reidenberg, M. (1996) 'Barriers to controlling pain in patients with cancer', Commentary, *The Lancet*, **347**(May 11): 1278.

Relf, M. (1989) *The Evaluation of a Bereavement Service: Some Early Reflections*, Association of Hospice Social Workers Annual Conference, September 1989, Oxfordshire: Milton.

Relf, M. (1995) 'Bereavement' in Twycross R. (ed.) *Introducing Palliative Care*, Oxford: Radcliffe.

Relf, M. and Couldrick, A. (1988) 'Bereavement support: the relationship between professionals and volunteers' in Gilmore, A. and Gilmore, S. (eds) *A Safer Death: Multi-disciplinary Aspects of Terminal Care*, New York: Plenum Press.

Rosenfield, M. and Urben, L. (1994) *Running a Telephone Cancer Support Group*, London: Cancerlink.

Royle, J. A. et al. (1996) The research utilization process: the use of guided imagery to reduce anxiety, *Canadian Oncology Nursing Journal*, 6(1): 20–25.

Rutter, D. R. (1987) *Communicating by Telephone*, Oxford: Pergamon Press.

Salamagne, M. and Keunebroek, N. (1996) 'Catering for the needs of foreign patients', *European Journal of Palliative Care*, 3(1): 32–34.

Schut, H. A. W. et al. (1997) 'Intervention for the bereaved: Gender differences in the efficacy of two counselling programmes', *British Journal of Clinical Psychology*, **36**: 63–72.

Schwab, R. (1996) 'Gender differences in parental grief', *Death Studies*, **20**(2): 103–113.

Scrutton, S. (1996) 'What can you expect, my dear, at my age?: recognising the need for counselling in a residential unit', *Bereavement Care*, **15**(3): 28–9.

Seale, C. (1991) 'Death from cancer and other causes: the relevance of the hospice approach', *Palliative Medicine*, **5**(1): 12–19.

Seale, C. and Cartwright, A. (1994) *The Year before Death*, Aldershot: Avebury.

Sheldon, F. (1997) *Psychosocial Palliative Care: Good Practice in the Care of the Dying and Bereaved*, Cheltenham: Stanley Thornes.

Sherr, L. (ed.) (1995) *Grief and AIDS*, Chichester: Wiley.

Silverman, P. R. and Worden, J. W. (1993) 'Children's reactions to the death of a parent', in Stroebe, M. S., Hansson, R. O. and Stroebe, W. (eds) *The Handbook of Bereavement: Theory, Research and Intervention*, Cambridge: Cambridge University Press.

Slevin, M. L. et al. (1988) 'BACUP – the first two years: evaluation of a national cancer information service', *British Medical Journal*, **297**: 669–672.

SMAC and SNMAC (1992) *The Principles and Provision of Palliative Care. Joint report of the Standing Medical Advisory Committee and Standing Nursing and Midwifery Advisory Committee*, London: HMSO.

Smaje, C. and Field, D. (1997) 'Absent minorities? Ethnicity and the use of palliative care services' in Field, D., Hockey, J. and Small, N. (eds) *Death, Gender and Ethnicity*, London: Routledge.

Smith, A. (1994) 'Review of palliative medicine education for medical students', *Medical Education*, **28**: 197–99.

Smith, A. (1996) 'Continuing education and short courses', *Palliative Medicine*, **10**(2): 105–111.

Smith, A. and Eve, A. M. (1994) 'Palliative care services in Britain and Ireland' *Palliative Medicine*, 8(1): 19–27.

Smith, N. (1990) 'The impact of terminal illness on the family', *Palliative Medicine*, 4: 127–135.

Smith, N. and Regnard, C. (1993) 'Managing family problems in advanced disease – a flow diagram', *Palliative Medicine*, 7: 47–58.

Smith, S. and Pennells, M. (eds) (1995) *Interventions with Bereaved Children*, London: Kingsley.

Spiegel, D. et al. (1989) 'Effect of psychosocial treatment on survival of patients with metastatic breast cancer', *Lancet*, 14 October, 2(668): 888–91.

St Christopher's Hospice Information Service (1994) *A Bereavement Care Team. Fact Sheet No. 22*, October, London: St Christopher's Hospice.

Stanway, A. (1995) *Sexuality and Cancer*, London: BACUP.

Stewart, J. and Paddle, A. (1994) *Guidelines for Setting up a Bereavement Counselling and Support Service*, London: National Association of Bereavement Services.

Stokes, J. and Crossley, D. (1995) 'Camp Winston. A residential intervention for bereaved children' in Smith, S. and Pennells, M. (eds) *Interventions with Bereaved Children*. London: Kingsley.

Stokes, J., Wyer, S. and Crossley, D. (1997) 'The challenge of revaluating a child bereavement programme', *Palliative Medicine*, 11(3): 179–190.

Stoller, R. (1968) *Sex and Gender*, New York: Science House.

Stroebe, M. (1996) 'Sex differences in bereavement', *Progress in Palliative Care*, 4: 85–87.

Stroebe, M., Stroebe, W. and Hansson, R. (eds) (1993) *Handbook of Bereavement Theory, Research and Intervention*, Cambridge: Cambridge University Press.

Telephone Helplines Association (1993), *Guidelines for Good Practice*, London: THA.

Townsend, J. et al. (1990) 'Terminal cancer care and patients' preference for place of death: a prospective study', *British Medical Journal*, **301** (1 September): 415–417.

Toynbee, Polly (1996), *Radio Times*, 10–16 August.

Twycross, R. (1995) *Introducing Palliative Care*, Oxford: Radcliffe.

Urben, L. (1997) 'Self-help groups in palliative care', *European Journal of Palliative Care*, 4(1): 26–28.

Vachon, M. L. S. (1995) 'Stress in hospice/palliative care: a review', *Palliative Medicine*, 9(2): 91–122.

Venn, M. J. et al. (1996) 'The experience and impact of contacting a cancer information service', *European Journal of Cancer Care*, 5(1): 38–42.

Vincent, C. E., et al. (1975) 'Some marital concomitants of carcinoma of the cervix', *South Med. Journal*, 68: 552–8.

Wallbank, S. (1992) *The Empty Bed. Bereavement and the Loss of Love*, London: Darton, Longman and Todd.

Walsh, F. and McGoldrick, M. (1991) 'Loss of the family: a systemic perspective' in Walsh, F. and McGoldrick, M. (eds) *Living Beyond Loss. Death in the Family*, New York: Norton.

Walter, T. (1996) 'A new model of grief: bereavement and biography', *Mortality* 1(1): 7–25.

Wilkes, E. (1993) 'Characteristics of hospice bereavement services', *Journal of Cancer Care*, 2:183–189.

Williams, M. (1996a) 'Men and bereavement', *Lifeline, The Newsletter of the National Association of Bereavement Services*, Autumn/Winter, 21: 9–11.

Williams, M. (1996b) 'Men and grief', Paper given to Tenth Annual Conference of the Association of Hospice and Specialist Palliative Care Social Workers. September, Glasgow.

Williams, M. (1997) 'Listening to men's voices: engaging and talking with male visitors to patients on hospice wards', MSc paper in preparation.

Winston's Wish (1995) A grief support programme for children *Progress report 1993–1995*, Gloucester: Winston's Wish.

Worden, W. J. (1991) *Grief Counselling and Grief Therapy*, 2nd edn, London: Tavistock Publications.

World Health Organization (1986) *Concepts of Sexual Health*, Regional Office for Europe. Eur./Mch.S21, Copenhagen: WHO.

World Health Organization (1990), *Cancer Pain Relief and Palliative Care. Technical Report 804*, Geneva: World Health Organization.

Yalom, I. D. (1995) *The Theory and Practice of Group Psychotherapy*, 4th edition, New York: Basic Books.

Index